improve
your eyesight
naturally

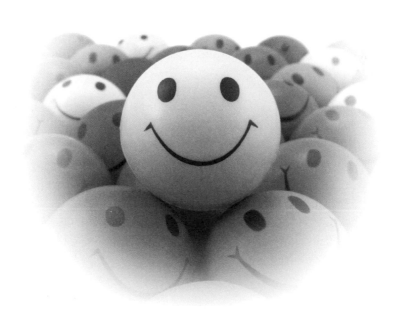

Leo Angart

improve
your eyesight
naturally

see results quickly

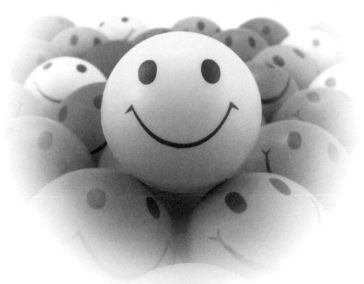

Crown House Publishing Limited
www.crownhouse.co.uk
www.crownhousepublishing.com

First published by

Crown House Publishing Ltd
Crown Buildings, Bancyfelin, Carmarthen,
Wales, SA33 5ND, UK
www.crownhouse.co.uk

and

Crown House Publishing Company LLC
6 Trowbridge Drive, Suite 5, Bethel, CT 06801, USA
www.crownhousepublishing.com

Cartoons © Göçhen Eke 2004, 2012
Anatomical drawings © Amass Communications Ltd. 2004, 2012
Smiley ball image © Uros Petrovic - Fotolia.com

Originally printed in paperback (ISBN: 9783937553085)

British Library Cataloguing-in-Publication Data
A catalogue entry for this book is available
from the British Library.

Print ISBN 978-184590801-0
Mobi ISBN 978-184590808-9
ePub ISBN 978-18459009-6
LCCN 2011938904

Printed and bound in the UK by, Bell & Bain Ltd, Glasgow

DISCLAIMER

Improve your Eyesight Naturally is not meant for diagnosis and treatment for any medical condition for the eye or
the visual system. The author, publisher and distributor are in no way liable for any damage whatsoever arising
from the use or misuse of this material or the exercises suggested including but not limited to any personal injury.
If you are in any doubt contact your doctor.

I would like to dedicate this book to my special star, Rebecca Szeto, who has provided many valuable suggestions and has been a great support during the writing of this book.

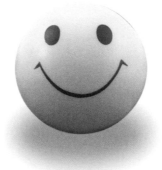

Acknowledgments

I wish to thank Dr. William H. Bates for his courage and determination in following his convictions and thus building the foundations upon which Vision Training rests.

I also wish to thank Master Choa Kok Sui for his dedication in developing the pranic healing approach. It was pranic healing that cured my eyesight. I realized early on that energy is a key factor if you want to have consistent success in regaining your eyesight.

A heartfelt thank you to my NLP trainers – John Grinder for inspiring me to start this adventure, and Judith DeLozier and Robert Dilts for teaching me to look for *the difference that makes the difference*. My approach is built on NLP methodology.

A special thank you goes to my dedicated sponsors, in particular Katrina Patterson in London, who encouraged me to put all this knowledge into a book. I also want to thank Lulu Heinse in Ireland and Monika and Maurice Cruz first in Manila and now in Melbourne for inviting me. Also a thank you to Wolfgang Gillessen in Munich for his valuable input in making the German version of this book a reality.

My proofreader put in long hours to make my manuscript much more enjoyable to read. Thank you to Candice Temple.

Finally, I want to thank the many people who attended my workshops and benefited from what they learned and I thank you for reading and benefiting from this book.

Contents

Acknowledgments i

1. **Introduction** **1**

2. **How to Benefit From This Book** **5**
   What is Vision Training? 6
   A brief history of Vision Training 8

3. **Regaining Your Eyesight – Is It Possible?** **15**
   Have your eyes tested 16
   Visiting the optometrist 17
   Understanding your prescription 18

4. **Anatomy of the Eye** **21**
   The eye muscles 21
   The cornea 23
   Optimal dimensions of the eye 25
   The lens 26
   The retina 28
   Photosensitive cells 29
   The macula 30

5. **Healthy Eyes** **33**
   What's needed for optimum eye health? 33
   What can I do to maintain optimum eye health? 34

6. **Visual Acuity** **39**
   Detecting small changes in visual acuity 40
   Night vision 43
   Contrast 44

What is a diopter? 45

7. Vision: The Mind Side **47**
It's a wonderful world out there 48
Where does your attention go? 49
Sensory alignment excercise 50

8. The Basic Principles of Vision Training **55**
Updating your beliefs about vision 62
Your reality strategy 62
Your belief strategy 64
The belief change cycle 67

9. Exercise Your Ability to See **69**
How to discover your internal vision 70
Find your dominant eye 70
Balancing your imaginary and physical vision 71
Are you avoiding what you don't want to see? 72

10. Getting Energy to Flow **75**
Chinese acupressure for your eyes 77

11. Check Your Eyesight **81**
Relax and see 81
How to test your distance vision 82
How to check if your myopia is more than 4 diopters 83
Near vision test 87

12. Astigmatism **89**
Vision Training principles for astigmatism 90
Exercise to loosen the eye muscles 93
Tibetan wheel exercise 94
Some objective proof 96

13. Myopia **99**
What causes myopia? 99

14. Recovering Myopia of Less Than 2 Diopters **109**
How to practice with the eye-chart 110
Swinging 111

15. Recovering Myopia from between 2 to 3 Diopters **113**

Chart-shifting exercise 114

The domino exercise 116

16. Recovering More Than 4 Diopters of Myopia **119**

Energy exercise 121

String exercise 124

Coming and going exercise 126

17. Presbyopia **129**

Bates' road to discovering the cure for presbyopia 131

Stumbling on the truth 132

Vision Training principles for presbyopia 133

Do you have presbyopia? 136

Small print exercise 136

Lazy reading exercise 141

Circle exercise 142

18. Hyperopia **145**

Vision Training principles for hyperopia 146

19. Convergence **149**

Vision Training principles for convergence 150

How to test for convergence 151

Convergence and reading 152

Convergence practice exercise 153

20. Strabismus **155**

How to test for strabismus 158

Vision Training principles for strabismus 159

The butterfly exercise 160

The long body swing exercise 161

The mirror swing exercise 162

The balance swing exercise 163

Tromboning exercise 164

21. Amblyopia **167**

Vision Training principles for amblyopia 169

22. Color Perception **171**
   Opponent color theory 172
   Hue discrimination 173
   Color perception deficiency 174
   Counting colors 176
   Matching colors 177
   Working with colors 177

23. The Visually Impaired **181**
   Gaining light perception 182
   Relaxing your eyes 182
   Mapping across your senses 182
   Gaining object recognition 183

24. Beyond 20/20 Vision **185**
   Exercise to improve distance vision 182

25. Mono-Vision **189**

26. Sunglasses **191**

27. Surgical Eyes **195**

28. Your Vision Training Plan **201**

Appendix: The Science of Vision Training 205

Bibliography 213

Index 223

About the Author 227

1. Introduction

Vision is the most precious of our senses. You see the splendor of a sunset, you see the smile on the face of someone you love and you see the innocence in the eyes of a child. Mother Nature has made certain that this sense is perfectly developed as we grow up. It may come as a surprise to you to hear that eyesight acuity is actually a skill we learn as we mature, and that the eyes of an infant are not fully developed. A baby begins to recognize colors at the age of about 4 months. Hand and eye co-ordination develop next and then co-ordination between eyes and body. At about 12 months of age babies begin to walk and from then on their vision continues to develop in the way that nature intended.

I am writing this book based on my own experience of wearing glasses for more than 25 years. Initially, like most people, I believed there was nothing that could be done about failing eyesight. It seemed that it was just a consequence of growing old – the only thing in question being whether hair or eyes would go first. At the time, 1991, my eyesight measured 5.5 diopters of near-sight. That means it was necessary for me to wear glasses for most things, including reading. In fact I needed two pairs of glasses, one for reading and another for distance.

A friend of mine had been working on improving his eyesight, but he had been trying for three years and was still wearing glasses. Long-term projects do not appeal to me. I like to feel that I am making progress in 20 minutes or less, otherwise I am not interested. I don't expect to have 20/20 vision after just one exercise, but I do want to sense that I am progressing and not just imagining that something is happening. So the approach I teach works fast.

In 1990 I became interested in something called neuro-linguistic programming (NLP). A seminal book in that field is *Trance-formations*, by Richard Bandler and John Grinder. The book is basically a transcript of a hypnosis seminar. On page 177 the authors describe a regression where they take a client back into their childhood. As we know, as children we generally have perfect eyesight. In a flash of inspiration,

Grinder brought the client back to the present, but with the eyesight of his childhood. Suddenly the client was able, as in his childhood, to see without glasses.

I was very excited about this. Imagine what it would be like if you could visit a hypnotherapist and emerge, after a mere hour, with perfect eyesight. Unfortunately, the universe had other ideas, since I could not find anyone who could lead me through this process. However, my interest was aroused because I concluded that there must be a way of regaining one's eyesight naturally.

Initially I played around with visualization exercises and they helped to a degree. However, I wanted to be completely cured and altogether eliminate the need for lenses. So I continued my quest for a way to recover my innate natural vision.

One Friday night I was going through the books I had acquired and happened to pick up one about healing with energy. In this book there was an exercise that was supposed to be good for near-sight. So I tried it and immediately felt that my eyes were becoming stronger. I continued doing this exercise every two hours and, eureka, the next day, after lunch, I was able to read without glasses. I have never needed reading glasses since. Throughout the weekend I continued with the exercise and on Monday morning I decided to go to work without glasses. I took a train and, as far as I know, there were no accidents that day! I was determined to keep the glasses off until after lunch at least. By lunchtime my eyes were very tired. If you have a high degree of near-sight you will know that taking off your glasses makes your eyes feel weary very quickly. However, I continued practicing the energy exercise and was gradually able to keep the glasses off for longer and longer periods. By the end of the week I was able to manage without glasses for the whole day. From then on I kept the glasses in my pocket, only taking them out to use as a magnifying glass on the A–Z if I needed to pick up someone from the airport. I did not want my subconscious mind to get any ideas that I wasn't serious about this.

From then on my vision kept improving and after another two weeks I could recognize people on the other side of the street, so my social life picked up once again. I did nothing about my eyes for the next five years and more or less forgot that I had ever worn glasses. Then, in 1995, I attended a month-long NLP Master Practitioner training at the NLP University, Santa Cruz, California. During the program I mentioned to my friends that I used to wear glasses. They appeared to be very interested and urged me to tell them what I did to achieve this seemingly remarkable feat. So I planned an evening talk and no less than 60 people showed up. This was an eye-opener(!) for me. Until then I had not realized that so many people were interested in getting rid of their glasses.

The following year, 1996, I was back at the NLP University for another course. This time we were required to have a "modeling project" – some area of excellence that we could explore and then develop a way of transferring this knowledge to others. At the time I did not know anyone who had regained their eyesight so there was nobody I could ask to help me with this. I decided that I would model myself and use my own experience as the basis for a new approach to curing near-sight. At this time I started buying books on how to recover your eyesight, such as William Bates' *Seeing without Glasses* (1920) and Janet Goodrich's *Natural Vision Improvement* (1986). From these I learned about the techniques of palming, sunning and so on.

By this point, I had come to the conclusion that it was prudent to have an understanding of any underlying beliefs that could be getting in the way of having clear eyesight. This was probably because, by then, I had learned effective ways of regressing people back in time. I uncovered a lot of interesting information about the kinds of life experiences that could have an impact on one's eyesight. Mostly it boiled down to innocent conclusions made by the mind of a child. For example, one little boy was moved from one school to another as an 8-year-old and as a consequence he lost all his friends. Another child uncovered a memory about taking a dislike to a teacher. Some of the experiences involved people seeing things they were not supposed to see. Others concerned events happening in their lives that they did not like but were powerless to do anything about. When I first started putting workshops together, I was convinced that about half of those attending would need subsequent personal one-on-one sessions in order to help them to see their beliefs for what they are and become free of these limitations.

In the process of creating the workshops I started learning about other kinds of common vision problems. For example, at the time I had no idea what astigmatism was, much less what to do about it. In the process of learning about different conditions, I started figuring out what exercises could be of help.

Before the lunch break on the first workshop, one myopic participant found that he could read the 20/20 line on the eye-chart, as well as the small print. This was a great pat on the back and I realized that most of the participants could benefit from my program. Coincidences and small miracles kept occurring and I was invited to more and more places to present the workshop. Since 1996 I have presented about 25 workshops per year in cities around the world. For example, I have given the workshop more than 25 times in London. Often I meet people who tell me they had wanted to come to my workshop for years before an opportunity presented itself.

I prefer the workshop approach to one-on-one sessions. This is because in 14 hours you will experience and learn more about your eyesight than I can possibly teach in an hour. Group dynamics are helpful in encouraging and motivating people to go away and actually do the exercises. It is not only a matter of getting the information, but also about realizing that you have more power than you think over your own eyesight and that there are steps you can take to improve it. The intended outcome of the workshop is that participants will discover the fact that they have control over their own eyesight and will get to know exactly what exercises they have to do and what results to expect.

I do not intend to play down the amount of work that is needed, which in some cases will mean doing eye exercises for years. What I do promise is that you will experience progress – your eyes will show you that they can improve and change. Scientific research shows that your eyesight has improved if you can see and identify five letters one line lower than previously on the eye-chart. In my workshop many people report seeing three or even four lines lower at the end of the session. Incidentally, as you descend the eye-chart, each line that you drop represents a 5 percent improvement in visual acuity. Experiencing a 10 to 20 percent observable and measurable improvement in just two days is a considerable achievement. On one occasion, in Berlin, we had an optometrist measuring people's eyesight before and after the workshop. One woman's eyesight measured 2 diopters less on Sunday evening before she went home. What is remarkable about this lady is that she was 92 years old!

Children respond even more rapidly. I have often seen children regain their "magic eyes" in less than an hour of Vision Training. One such example was 8-year-old Max, who at the beginning had a prescription of 20/40 near-sight. After 20 minutes of exercises he came back to me and told me that he could now see the 20/16 line on the eye-chart. For a child under 10 years it is normal to be able to see the last line on the eye-chart. The following year I met Max again and checked his eyesight. He could still see the 20/16 line, so either he had an incredible memory or his eyesight had truly improved.

I am writing this book because I want people to know that it really is possible to regain one's eyesight. Another reason is that I would like to share my learning with the world so many more people can benefit. This message is especially important for children. There is no reason why children should be condemned to a life wearing glasses when, in most cases, they can easily regain natural clear sight using the methods of Vision Training. Introduced early on, this approach is highly effective and has the added advantage of being natural and showing permanent results.

2. How to Benefit From This Book

I am sure that you will want to go right to the chapter dealing with your vision problem. Go ahead and read the chapter and do the tests provided to determine your visual acuity. Then I suggest that you read the first part of the book, which outlines the background and the general principles of the method. If you are interested in the scientific basis for the efficacy of this approach then read the appendix at the back of the book, where I have summarized some of the most important research for each eye condition.

After familiarizing yourself with my approach, I then suggest you start experimenting with the exercises in the sections most applicable to you. You should start experiencing results quite quickly. It is of primary importance to monitor your progress. Positive feedback is very important in keeping you self-motivated. There are of course limitations to the information that can be conveyed in print. Eventually you may want to attend a workshop where you will benefit from the live interaction and discover exactly what your prescription is and what to do about it.

My approach is not only about transmitting the information contained in this book, but also about influencing and motivating you to succeed. Ultimately it is down to you and I am just providing you with the *how*.

The website www.vision-training.com contains additional information, as well as more detailed research that is only just referred to in this book.

You may find it difficult to accomplish all this just by reading about it. At some point I recommend that you attend a workshop so that you can find out about your eyesight through live experience.

What is Vision Training?

Vision Training is based on the simple fact that exercise has a beneficial effect on your health. It is common knowledge that if you exercise regularly your wellbeing will improve. Your doctor will tell you that walking for as little as 30 minutes every day will significantly improve both health and fitness.

The American Optometric Association (1988) notes that, "The efficacy of Vision Training in remediating occulomotor, accommodative, and binocular disorders has been substantiated in many studies." Yet many eye-care professionals are either directly opposed to or very skeptical about Vision Training, Vision Therapy or orthoptics. They simply do not see any alternative to glasses or refractive surgery.

In general, eye-care professionals are most comfortable with the medical model of immediate treatment of symptoms. This is done very effectively by fitting glasses or by laser surgery. However, wearing glasses does absolutely nothing for your myopia. The lenses correct the refractive error, but you will still have myopia and the associated risks (i.e., 60 percent higher risk of retinal detachment, glaucoma and macular degeneration).

Laser surgery is the latest development in the mechanical approach to vision problems. What happens is that the lens is carved onto your cornea. Since the cornea is only half a millimeter thick any surgery significantly weakens the tissue. This is an inevitable consequence of surgery. Subsequent complications may impair your vision. Furthermore, your night vision is likely to be severely diminished, so you may not be able to drive when it is dark. Legislation is under way in the United States and Canada that may prohibit people who have undergone laser surgery from driving at night. In Germany special contrast tests are one of the requirements for a driver's license. Many people who have undergone LASIK (laser assisted in situ keratomileusis) laser surgery fail that test and consequently cannot get a driver's license. Some people also discover that they need to wear reading glasses after laser surgery. So they are, in effect, switching from one pair of glasses to another.

Vision Training is process orientated and aims to make you aware of internal changes taking place. The success of a Vision Training program depends on developing optimum vision strategies and making them second nature. My approach is to empower you and motivate you to do brief periods of exercises that last for about five minutes, but very frequently – perhaps ten times a day. Frequent repetition seems to be necessary for permanent changes to take place. Just doing eye exercises once a week is not enough to develop any meaningful change in myopia.

For Vision Training to be effective there has to be a clearly defined method of measuring progress. Most people quickly lose interest if they don't perceive any improvement. Therefore it is important to make certain that progress is constantly noted and celebrated. A meaningful change in myopia would be a consistent decrease in measurement over a period of time.

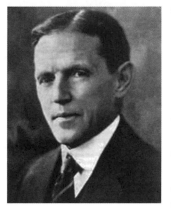

The grandfather of Vision Training

Dr. William Bates graduated from the College of Physicians and Surgeons, Columbia University in 1885.

From 1886 to 1896 Dr. Bates was Assistant Surgeon at the New York Eye and Ear Infirmary, North-Western Dispensary and Harlem Hospital. Bates was also an instructor in ophthalmology at the New York Post-Graduate Medical School and Hospital. He was a successful and well-respected eye surgeon. However, he taught medical students how to improve their near-sightedness and as a consequence was expelled from the faculty in 1891.

Dr. Bates published many papers in the *New York Medical Journal* about his discovery that eyesight problems are learned and functional. As a result he believed that the eyes are responsive to exercises that involve relaxation.

Bates developed a series of simple exercises designed for various vision problems. He published his work in a *New York Medical Journal* article, "The Cure of Defective Eyesight by Treatment without Glasses" in 1915. The work was later re-edited and published as *Better Eyesight without Glasses* (1940). The book is still available today.

William Bates is considered by many to be the grandfather of Vision Training.

A brief history of Vision Training

The idea that one can train the eyes with exercise originates with New York ophthalmologist William H. Bates, M.D. (1860–1931). Dr. Bates examined thousands of eyes every year as part of his work at the New York Eye and Ear Infirmary. Over the years he began to question the wisdom of the theories put forward by the founding fathers of ophthalmology.

> Examining 30,000 pairs of eyes a year at the New York Eye and Ear Infirmary and other institutions, I observed many cases in which errors of refraction either recovered spontaneously, or changed their form, and I was unable either to ignore them, or to satisfy myself with the orthodox explanations, even where such explanations were available. It seemed to me that if a statement is truth it must always be truth. There can be no exceptions. If errors of refraction are irreversible, they should not recover nor change their form spontaneously.

> In the course of time I discovered that myopia and hypermetropia, like astigmatism, could be produced at will; that myopia was not, as we have so long believed, associated with the use of the eyes at the near point, but with a strain to see distant objects, strain at the near point being associated with hypermetropia; that no error of refraction was ever a constant condition. (Bates, 1920: 12)

At the time a new instrument, the retinoscope invented by the eminent German scientist Hermann von Helmholtz (1821–1894), became available. The focusing ability of the eye can be determined by observing it through this instrument. Dr. Bates examined the eyes of his patients in all sorts of conditions and thus learned a great deal about the way they focus.

> Much of my information about the eyes has been obtained by means of simultaneous retinoscopy. The retinoscope is an instrument used to measure the refraction of the eye. It throws a beam of light into the pupil by reflection from a mirror, the light being outside the instrument either – above and behind – the subject is arranged within it by means of an electric battery. On looking through the retinoscope one sees a larger or smaller part of the pupil filled with light. In normal human eyes this would be a reddish yellow, the color of the retina, but could be white if the retina is diseased. In a cat's eye it would be green. Unless the eye is exactly focussed at the point from which it is being observed, one would see a dark shadow at the edge of the pupil. It is the behaviour of this shadow, when the mirror is moved in various directions, which reveals the refractive condition of the eye ... This exceedingly useful instrument has possibilities which have not been generally realized by the medical profession ...

For thirty years I have been using the retinoscope to study the refraction of the eye. With it I have examined the eyes of tens of thousands of school children, hundreds of infants and thousands of animals, including cats, dogs, rabbits, horses, cows, birds, turtles, reptiles and fish. I have used it when the subjects were at rest and when they were in motion – also when I myself was in motion. I have used it in daytime and at night, when the subjects were comfortable and when they were excited; when they were trying to see and when they were not; when they were lying and when they were telling the truth; when the eyelids were partly closed, shutting off part of the area of the pupil, when the pupil was dilated, and also when it was contracted to a pin-point; when the eyes were oscillating from side to side, from above downward and in other directions. In this way I discovered many facts, which had not previously been known, and which I was quite unable to reconcile with the orthodox teachings on the subject. This led me to undertake the series of experiments already alluded to. The results were in entire harmony with my previous observations, and left me no choice but to reject the entire body of orthodox teachings about accommodation and refraction. (Bates, 1920: 17)

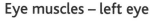

Eye muscles – left eye

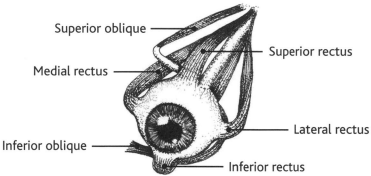

Superior oblique

Superior rectus

Medial rectus

Inferior oblique

Lateral rectus

Inferior rectus

One thing that became clear to Bates early on was that the eyes are in a constant state of change. If you were to measure them every hour each measurement would be slightly different. Dr. Bates' discoveries are almost directly opposite to conventional thinking about the way the eye focuses. Donders (1864) and later Helmholtz (1866) concluded that it was mainly the lens inside the eye that did the focusing. This theory still prevails today and greatly influences eye-care professionals. Again, in Bates' own words:

The function of the muscles on the outside of the eyeball, apart from that of turning the globe in its socket, has been a matter of much dispute; but after the supposed demonstration by Helmholtz that accommodation depends on the change in curvature of the lens, the possibility of their being concerned in the adjustment of the eye for vision at different distances, or in the production of errors of refraction, was dismissed as no longer worthy of serious consideration ... In my own experiments upon the extrinsic eye muscles of fish, rabbits, cats, dogs and other animals, the demonstration seemed to suggest that in the eyes of these animals accommodation depends wholly upon the action of the extrinsic muscles and not at all upon the agency of the lens. By manipulation of these muscles I was able to produce or prevent accommodation at will, to myopia, hypermetropia and astigmatism, or to prevent these conditions. Full details of these experiments will be found in the "Bulletin of the New York Zoological Society" for November, 1914, and in the "New York Medical Journal" for May 8, 1915; and May 18, 1918; but for the benefit of those who have not the time or inclination to read these papers, their contents are summarized below.

There are six muscles on the outside of the eyeball, four known as the recti and two as the *obliques*. The obliques form an almost complete belt around the middle of the eyeball, and are known, according to their position, as superior and inferior. The recti are attached to the sclerotic, or outer coat of the eyeball, near the front, and pass directly over the top, bottom and sides of the globe to the back of the orbit, where they are attached to the bone around the edges of the hole through which the optic nerve passes. According to their position, they are known as the superior, inferior, internal, and external recti. The obliques are the muscles of accommodation; the recti are concerned in the production of hypermetropia and astigmatism.

In some cases one of the obliques is absent or rudimentary, but when two of these muscles were present and active, accommodation, as measured by the objective test of retinoscopy, was always produced by electrical stimulation either of the eyeball, or the nerves of accommodation near their origin in the brain. It was produced by any manipulation of the obliques whereby their pull was increased. This was done by a tucking operation of one or both muscles, or by an advancement of the point at which they are attached to the sclerotic. When one or more of the recti had been cut, the effect of operations increasing the pull of the obliques was intensified.

After one or both of the obliques had been cut across, or after they had been paralysed by the injection of atropine deep into the orbit, accommodation could never be produced by electrical stimulation; but after the effects of the atropine has passed away, or a divided muscle had been sewn together, accommodation followed electrical stimulation just as usual. Again, when one oblique muscle was absent, as was found to be the case in a dogfish, a shark and a few perch, or rudimentary, as in all cats observed, a few fish and an occasional rabbit, accommodation could not be produced by electrical stimulation. But when the rudimentary muscles were strengthened by advancement, or the absent one was replaced by a suture, which supplied the necessary counter traction, accommodation could always be produced by electrical stimulation.

It should be emphasized that in order to paralyse either the recti muscles, or the obliques, it was found necessary to inject the atropine far back behind the eyeball with a hypodermic needle. This drug is supposed to paralyse the accommodation when dropped into the eyes of human beings or animals, but in all of my experiments it was found that when used in this way it had very little effect upon the power of the eye to change its focus.

...

Eyes from which the lens had been removed, or in which it had been pushed out of the axis of vision, responded to electrical stimulation precisely as did the normal eye, so long as the muscles were active; but when they had been paralysed by the injection of atropine deep into the orbit, electrical stimulation had no effect on the refraction.

In one experiment the lens was removed from the right eye of a rabbit, the refraction of each eye having first been tested by retinoscopy and found to be normal. The wound was then allowed to heal. Thereafter, for a period extending from one month to two years, electrical stimulation always produced accommodation in the lensless eye precisely to the same extent as in the eye which had a lens. The same result was performed on a number of other rabbits, on dogs and on fish. The obvious conclusion is that the lens is not a factor in accommodation.

In most text-books on physiology it is stated that accommodation is controlled by the third cranial nerve, which supplies all the muscles of the eyeball except the superior oblique and the external rectus; both the fourth cranial nerve, which supplies only the superior oblique, was found in these experiments to be just as much a nerve of accommodation as the third.

When either the third or the fourth nerve was stimulated with electricity near its point of origin in the brain, accommodation always resulted in the normal eye. When the origin of either nerve was covered with a small wad of cotton soaked in a two percent solution of atropine sulphate in a normal salt solution, stimulation of that nerve produced no accommodation, while stimulation of the unparalysed nerve did produce accommodation. When the origin of both nerves was covered with cotton soaked in atropine, accommodation could not be produced by electrical stimulation of either or both nerves. When the cotton was removed and the nerves washed with normal salt solution, electrical stimulation of either or both produced accommodation just as before the atropine had been applied. This experiment, which was performed repeatedly for more than an hour by alternately applying and removing the atropine, not only demonstrated clearly what had not been known before, namely, that the fourth nerve is a nerve of accommodation, but also demonstrated that the superior oblique muscle which is supplied by it, is an important factor in accommodation. It was further found that when the action of the oblique muscles was prevented by dividing them, the stimulation the of third nerve produced not accommodation but hypermetropia. (Bates, 1920: 38–45)

Dr. Bates' discovery was not met with great enthusiasm by the scientific community. In fact he was unceremoniously dismissed from his teaching post at the New York Eye and Ear Infirmary. The internal power structure found his views too radical a departure from the then accepted scientific norm. However, Bates went on to develop his theory on his own and established a clinic where Vision Training was available. He also published a magazine called *Better Eyesight* and trained a number of people in the techniques he developed.

Today we know Bates' work as the "Bates Method," which he outlined in his book *Better Eyesight without Glasses*. The interest in Vision Training has endured to this day and Bates' book is still in print more than 80 years after its original publication.

Since then the scientific community, with only a few exceptions, has completely ignored Bates' findings. The proponents of the Bates Method have been people who were helped by the technique.

One such person was Margaret D. Corbett whose husband was greatly helped by the Bates Method in the 1930s. Mrs. Corbett went on to establish the School of Eye Education in Los Angeles and trained many people in the Bates Method. In her book *Help Yourself to Better Sight* (1949) she describes many incidents where her work had great impact on the careers of military men. One such story concerns a young man who had been rejected several times by the Air Force because of deficient vision. He normalized his eyes by using the Bates exercises, passed all tests and joined the Flying Tigers in Burma where he became a flight leader. He returned with ten Japanese planes to his credit. After that, his score continued to mount, as did his rank, and he eventually became a lieutenant colonel.

In 1955 Clara Hackett published *Relax and See: A Daily Guide to Better Vision*. The book is designed around a 12-week exercise program for various vision problems.

These include the common problems like myopia and hyperopia, plus exercises for bifocal wearers, crossed eyes, color-blindness and cataracts as well as glaucoma and serious vision problems. She also included step-by-step exercises for the blind.

Miss Hackett, who herself wore glasses for more than 19 years, taught eye training in Seattle for five years and trained teachers under the G.I. Bill of Rights. She was on the visiting faculty of Seattle University in 1949 and 1950, giving courses in Vision Training. After moving to New York, she was arrested in 1950 on the charge of practicing optometry without a license and appeared before a grand jury in 1951. The jury deliberated only for few minutes – Vision Training is not a crime.

Janet Goodrich, Ph.D., in discussing possible reasons why so few people have heard of the Bates Method, writes:

> [T]he professional, technically trained eye practitioners ... were taught that the Bates method was ineffective, to be derided and disdained ...

> Margaret Corbett admonished the hundreds of teachers she trained in the 1940s and 1950s never to advertise, lecture, or publish articles. More understanding is generated by the knowledge that she was arrested (and acquitted) twice for practicing optometry without a license ...

> In 1974, my colleague in San Francisco, Mrs. Anna Kaye, who'd been quietly transmitting Bates Method principles for several decades, was visited by undercover agents. She was told she was breaking the law on sixteen counts ...

> You may now realize why substantiated objective proof is scarce. (1986: 184–185)

Goodrich contributed greatly to the field of Vision Training through her two books Natural Vision Improvement (1986) and *Perfect Sight the Natural Way* (1996), as well as her lectures and workshops around the world.

In 1997 Thomas R. Quackenbush published *Relearning to See*, which is perhaps the most comprehensive book on the Bates Method to date. The book adheres very closely to Bates' original work and Quackenbush often quotes Bates' publications extensively. Thomas Quackenbush is based in Holland.

Indian ophthalmologist Dr. R. S. Agarwal became interested in Bates' work in 1930 and has since been actively teaching the Bates Method in Pondicherry in India. Over the years Agarwal published many articles in *Mother India*, a monthly journal of the Sri Aurobindo Ashram, as well as developing a synthesis of traditional ophthalmology and the Bates Method which was published in *Mind and Vision and Secrets of Indian Medicine*. A popular book called *Yoga of Perfect Eyesight* was published in 1971.

This book is still in print and contains many wonderful stories of how Dr. Agarwal helped people regain their eyesight.

In the U.K. the Bates Method has taken root and is represented by the Bates Association of Great Britain. The method is described in *The Bates Method* by Peter Mansfield (1997).

During the 1990s there was a marked movement towards complementary approaches in dealing with health problems. For example, acupuncture was accepted as a valid treatment method and is now taught in several medical schools.

However, the economic advantages of prescribing drugs or devices is financially much more lucrative than simply training the eyes to regain their normal state of clear vision. Even more lucrative is recommending refractive surgery, which costs thousands of dollars per eye.

From the consumer's point of view, the most effective way to treat the problem is not necessarily the most expensive way. Hopefully the new millennium will see an increased interest in effective, non-invasive methods by people in general and by science in particular. Currently the percentage of people wearing glasses is almost 60 percent of the general population. In Asia this figure is fast approaching 80 percent of the population. Something needs to be done to put it right.

Vision Training, started early on, is the simple answer to maintaining good eyesight.

3. Regaining Your Eyesight – Is It Possible?

Most people believe that there is nothing you can do about deteriorating vision. The prevailing wisdom is that as we grow older our senses begin to fail and eyesight just happens to be the one that tends to go first.

Scientists tell us that statistically the world's population of 6-year-olds has bright and clear vision. A study of myopia (near-sight) over the last hundred years commissioned by the U.S. Army, tells us that the prevalence of vision problems is currently around 60 percent.

Eye doctors (ophthalmologists) learn virtually nothing about Vision Training when they attend medical school. The focus is on the use of drugs and surgery. Indeed, surgery is the proffered solution for many serious eye problems. Lenses are the most common remedy suggested, with laser surgery recommended if near-sight has been stable for at least three years. It is important to realize that wearing glasses does absolutely nothing for your near-sight. When you take off your glasses you are still near-sighted. The glasses do indeed provide a quick fix for the problem but they do not address the underlying reason you became near-sighted in the first place.

Laser surgery is currently very popular and is highly recommended by many ophthalmologists. Having the lenses carved on your cornea is an irrevocable way of altering your vision. However, all laser surgery actually does is shave a few microns off your cornea. Any mistake will be with you for the rest of your life. My eyes are the last place I want anyone to tinker, especially when there are natural ways of regaining one's eyesight. Optometrists are licensed and trained to measure your eyes and to prescribe corrective lenses. Their entire training revolves around the correction of visual defects and the selling of glasses. It is understandable, therefore, that they are not too enthusiastic about any suggestions that you can do away with your glasses altogether by simple Vision Training exercises.

Behavioural optometrists are a group who believe that exercises can reduce the progression of near-sightedness. They are generally open to the idea of Vision Training and will, in most cases, be happy to prescribe lenses lower than 100 percent correction. If you go to your optometrist or ophthalmologist and say that you want to do some Vision Training with the objective of getting rid of your glasses, you will most probably be told, very patiently, that this is unfortunately not possible and that you should continue to wear them.

Of all the optometrists practicing in Europe there are only about 200 who are members of various behavioural optometrist associations (The College of Optometrists in Vision Development (COVD) in the U.S. The British Association of Behavioural Optometrists (BABO) and Australasian College of Behavioural Optometrists (ACBO).

Functional or behavioural optometrists are mainly concerned with the treatment of amblyopia, strabismus and eye co-ordination problems. They do not yet have any methods for treating common visual problems such as astigmatism, myopia and hyperopia. The therapy approach usually involves an initial eye examination where your visual status is determined. Reduced lens prescription and eye exercises are then prescribed. Lately computer-aided Vision Training software has been developed and introduced. I have some reservations about this approach since computer work is one of the causes of myopia. Using the computer to eliminate vision problems seems to be a contradiction. Behavioural optometrists often use an assortment of equipment for measurement and training. My approach does not involve any mechanical equipment. There is nothing you need to buy or take; there are no expensive therapy sessions you need to pay for. What is required is your active participation by doing the appropriate exercises, and then you will see constant progress towards regaining your natural clear eyesight.

Have your eyes tested

There are two tests employed in determining what strength of lenses you need to correct your vision to perfect 20/20. Usually the optometrist will use a machine to get an objective reading. The machine employs a calculated average with a plus or minus half diopter margin of error. It tests for absolutely perfect focusing at a distance of 6 meters.

The second test is a subjective test where you look through several kinds of lenses in order to establish which ones are the most comfortable. This test usually takes place in a room with dim light. Part of the problem is that your eyes keep trying to adapt to the various lenses and in doing so you tend to be handed a prescription that is too strong. You have probably experienced coming back the next day and trying on the new glasses only to find that they hurt your eyes. This is because the glasses are over-corrected and the focus is too sharp for your eyes.

The human eye varies by as much as 2 diopters in visual acuity during the day. If you measure your vision every few hours you will discover a different reading every time.

However, it is a good idea to have your eyes tested before you start on your Vision Training program. You will then know precisely what the status of your vision is and how it will register on the eye doctor's equipment. Then go ahead and start your Vision Training. You will probably notice an improvement quite quickly. This is your subjective experience of vision which is always ahead of the objective measure. You might be able to actually see and read four or five more lines on the eye-chart, but the machine will not show any improvement at all. The machine measures only absolutely perfect focusing – not the fact that you can see better. Do yourself a favor and carry on with your Vision Training exercises for about a month before you go for another eye test. However, during that period you may need to have the power of your lenses reduced, since the old prescription will no longer be relevant and the lenses may start to hurt your eyes.

Visiting the optometrist

Some optometrists are opposed to reducing a prescription to less than the results of their test. If your optometrist belongs to that category, then I suggest you find someone else!

Let the optometrist measure your eyes using his instruments. By the way, just measuring your eyes with the automatic equipment is only a rough estimate. The machines vary and have a plus–minus error factor of half a diopter (one line on the eye-chart). When the optometrist has finished his test you will have what he determines to be 100 percent correction of your vision. Usually you will find this to be incredibly sharp and in some cases so sharp it actually hurts the eyes. Ask the optometrist to reduce the prescription by 0.5 or 1 diopter. Then go outside into the street and look though the test lenses he has prescribed. It is not enough to just look around in the optometry shop or the shopping mall. You need to see how the glasses work in daylight and by looking at the real world.

For the best results, get a prescription which gives you distance vision that is slightly soft. This will give a correction of about 20/40 distance vision. However, make sure that your prescription is not under-corrected by more than 1 diopter. If you reduce the correction more by than this there is a chance that you will actually begin to strain the eyes, in which case progress in Vision Training will be greatly reduced.

Optique 20/20	Date			Name		Tlf:		
Date:		Sph	Cyl	Axis	Prism	Add	Lens type	
Name:	Right	-2.50	0.50	85°				
I.D. No:								
Frame:	Left	11.50	-0.50	85°				
Lenses:								
Extras:								
Sub Total:	Contact Lenses	BC	Diam	Power	Solutions		Lens type	
C/L Consult:								
Total:								
Voucher:	Tint	Coating	Type	O.C.	Special instructions			
Deposit:								
Balance to pay:								
	Frame	Model	Size	Colour				

Understanding your prescription

The prescription you get from the optometrist looks like Greek to most people. It makes no sense whatsoever. Actually it is much simpler than it looks. Firstly it shows one measurement for the left eye and one for the right eye. Usually this is indicated with an "L" for the left eye and an "R" for the right.

The first column indicates the degree of refractive error (i.e., it tells you whether you are myopic and by what degree). This measurement is indicated in diopters. If you are myopic then there will be a minus indication such as -2.50 D – minus two-and-a-half diopters. In some countries this is referred to as 250 (they simply drop the period). If you are hyperopic (far-sighted) or presbyopic (need reading glasses) then the indication will be +1.50 D or plus one-and-a-half diopters. Note that there often is a difference in the prescription for each eye, as one eye is better than the other.

The next column indicates if there is any astigmatism. This is also measured in diopters as well as the axis in which the astigmatism is found. The notation might be something like this: Cyl: -0.5 Axis: 85. The translation reads a cylinder correction of minus one-half of a diopter at an 85 degree axis. Note it is possible to have astigmatism in only one eye, or that the degree and axis can differ from one eye to the other.

The third column is usually dedicated to divergence. The reading for strabismus is usually corrected using "prism elements." These are indicated in prism diopters and the Greek letter Δ is often used to indicate that a prism element is included.

There will generally be a space on the form for any additional notes from the optometrist. Sometimes near vision will also be tested, and there could be a prescription for combination or bifocal lenses. Another possibility is that you are given a prescription for glasses with variable focus lenses that have two or three areas with different lens power. Suggested lenses and frames are also often noted.

The slips of paper that are printed out from machines used to check visual acuity also show other numbers that are relevant if you are being fitted with contact lenses.

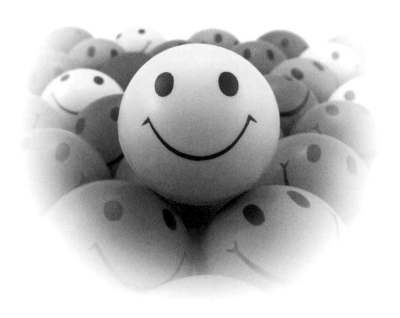

4. Anatomy of the Eye

The human eye is an anatomical masterpiece. The eye is about 24 mm in diameter and functions as the interface between the outside world and the inner world. The physical eye is responsible for capturing images of objects in the outer world. It is similar to a video camera and indeed they have many things in common. However, the human eye is far superior to any camera built to date. For example, the human eye has much greater sensitivity to light. You can find your way in almost complete darkness as well as deal with bright sunlight on a beach. The video camera has a very limited range in comparison to the human eye.

The eye muscles

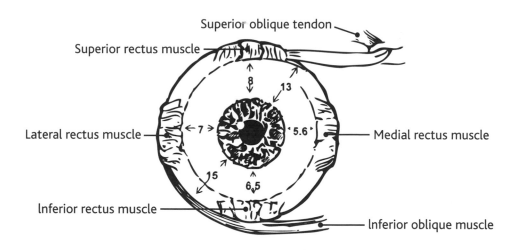

There are six external muscles attached to each eye. These muscles work in pairs to enable you to move your eyes in all directions. Eye muscles are unique in their ability to move the eye very quickly and precisely to point it in the direction of what you want to observe. The muscles can also adjust in real time and allow you to track a tennis ball from one end of a court to the other.

The four rectus muscles are located around the eye. The one above the eye – the rectus superior – is the muscle responsible for moving the eye upwards. The lower rectus muscle – the rectus inferior – is responsible for moving the eye downwards. These two muscles work in tandem to enable your eyes to move up and down to any degree. Horizontal movements of the eyes are accomplished by the medial rectus and lateral rectus muscles located on each side of the eye. Together the four rectus muscles give the eye the capacity to move in all directions.

In addition there is also a pair of muscles attached to the back of the eye. These are called the oblique muscles because they enable the eyes to move both towards and away from each other. This enables you to point your eyes as well as track objects moving towards and away from you. The upper – superior oblique – muscle is attached to the bone near the nose with a long tendon. This muscle is used when you cross your eyes towards your nose.

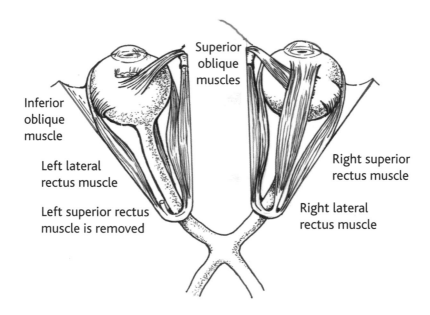

Your exterior eye muscles are also involved in adjusting the focus. In his pioneering research William H. Bates (1915) concluded that the oblique muscles focus by squeezing the eyeball and moving the retina into a position where the image is in perfect focus. He likened the function to that of a camera. When you want to focus it on something close-up, you move the lens forward. In the human eye the same principle is employed by squeezing the eyeball slightly to keep the image focused.

This action is mainly accomplished by the two oblique muscles. In myopia the back of the eye is permanently pushed out causing difficulty in focusing. Far-sight is a condition where the four rectus muscles are held very tightly causing the eyeball to become shorter. To give you an idea of the scale of these movements, each millimeter the eyeball is elongated is equivalent to approximately 3 diopters of myopia. With this degree of myopia your vision would go from normal to being able to see clearly only up to 30 cm, approximately the normal reading distance. The physical changes that take place are minute but with huge consequences.

Inside the eye there are two circular muscles. One muscle determines the size of the iris and how much light enters the eye. The other muscle is circular in shape and located around the lens.

The cornea

The clear part of the eye, the cornea, is responsible for about 75 percent of the focusing power of the eye. The greatest refractive effect is achieved at the interface between the air and the tear film. This is why refractive surgery is possible. Shaving off even minute portions of the cornea has a major effect on the focusing power of your eye.

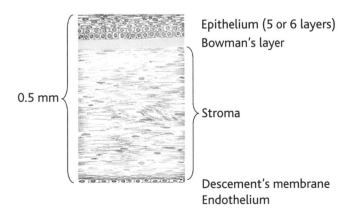

0.5 mm

Epithelium (5 or 6 layers)
Bowman's layer

Stroma

Descement's membrane
Endothelium

The cornea is about half a millimeter thick at the center of the pupil and consists of several layers. The outer layer is the tear film, which nourishes the cornea as well as being a part of the refractive elements of the eye. You have probably noticed that blinking your eyes improves your ability to see. The physical surface of the cornea is called the epithelium, which consists of a protective layer of relatively hard surface cells. Its function is to protect the eye from damage. Extended wearing of contact lenses, especially hard lenses, eventually wears down the corneal epithelium and contact lenses can no longer be worn.

Just a few cells below the surface we have Bowman's layer. This is a layer of collagen-like cells that help the cornea to keep its shape. This layer never heals if there has been a surgical intervention. Bowman's layer is like the stiffeners in your shirt collar. The largest part of the cornea is the stroma. This layer is where laser surgery is performed. Part of the stroma layer is blasted away in order to thin the cornea so that the refractive power will change. Since there are no blood vessels in the cornea it takes as much as six months to heal. Also there is an unavoidable weakening of the cornea due to the surgery.

Optical dimensions of the eye

This section is for those of you who are interested in the scientific aspects of the eye's optical dimensions. I am amazed that the eye is so small and that there are such huge differences in dioptric power between the cornea and the lens.

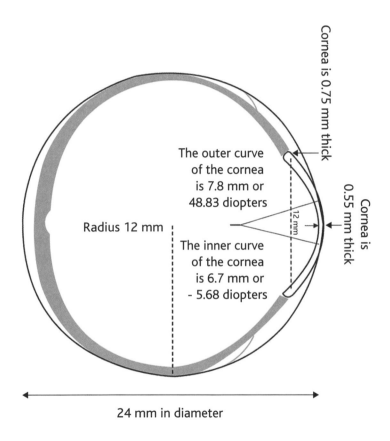

Eye structures	Average	Range
Refractive index		
Air	1.0	
Cornea	1.376	
Corneal epithelium	1.337	
Anterior corneal stroma	1.401	
Posterior corneal stroma	1.380	
Aqueous humor	1.373	
Vitreous humor	1.340	
Lens	1.336	
Central radius of curvature		
Anterior corneal surface	7.8 mm	7.0 – 8.6 mm
Posterior corneal surface	6.7 mm	
Diopter power		
Anterior corneal surface	49.50 diopters	39 – 48 diopters
Posterior corneal surface	-6.99 diopters	
Net corneal power	43.50 diopters	
Net lens power	20.00 diopters	
Total power of the eye	63.50 diopters	
Thickness		
Central cornea	0.56 mm	
Peripheral cornea	1.20 mm	
Corneal epithelium	0.06 mm	50 – 60 μm

The lens

While the cornea provides most of the optical power of the eye, the lens is an important part of the optical system. The lens is about 10 mm in diameter and consists of crystalline cells that are completely transparent so light can shine through.

The lens is suspended in space by tiny fibers called zonules. Because of its high water content the lens is very flexible and the pull of the zonules alters the shape of the lens. When the ciliary ring muscle is relaxed, the zonules are tightened and the lens becomes flatter – thus having less focusing power. On the other hand, when the ciliary muscle is contracted the zonules are relaxed and the lens bulges out and thus increases its focal power. When the ciliary muscle is relaxed the eye is said to have "accommodated."

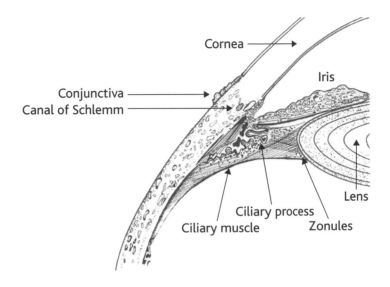

In vision tests, the drug atropine is sometimes used to paralyze the ciliary muscle. The rationale is that when ciliary muscle activity is eliminated you will then get the "true" visual status. Some optometrists believe that this is the only valid test. Applying the same logic, you might wonder why your spine is not paralyzed when its height is measured to eliminate the possibility that you will stretch up and become taller!

The crystalline cells of the lens remain the same throughout life. Each year a new layer grows like an onion. Between age 20 and 80 the lens will have doubled in thickness. The lens has no blood vessels and is therefore nourished only by the aqueous humor that is continuously secreted from the ciliary body. Vitamin C is the most important supplement for the lens. The lens has the highest concentration of vitamin C in the entire body. Oxidation damage by free radicals causes the crystalline cells in the lens to become opaque. This condition is known as cataracts. Since the lens is only a small part of the optical system of the eye, you can still see even if your lens has been removed – approximately 10 percent loss of visual acuity (or two lines on the eye-chart). Thus you could still be driving legally even without lenses in your eyes. The legal limit for driving is 20/40 visual acuity.

The retina

The retina is a paper-thin layer at the back of the eye which contains light sensitive cells. If the retina is damaged there will be permanent loss of vision. The most serious retina problems are macular degeneration and diabetic retinopathy, both of which are a form of deterioration of the integrity of the retina. Another problem is retinal detachment, which occurs in people with a high degree of myopia.

Light sensitivity

The trade-off between visual resolution and visual sensitivity is largely due to the way rod and cone cells are connected to the post-receptoral elements of the retina.

Rod cells are connected in such a way that they sum up information over space producing great sensitivity but poor resolution. Mother Nature achieves this by connecting many more rod cells in parallel to a single nerve fiber (ganglion cell). The scotopic vision manifests great spatial summation. On the other hand cone cell connections maximize visual resolution and the expanse of sensitivity.

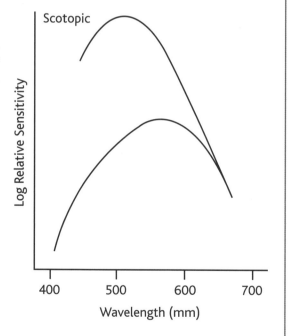

A ganglion cell requires ten quantal absorptions before it signals an event. Also the light must be present within a certain time frame, or it is lost.

Photosensitive cells

There are two kinds of photosensitive cells in the eyes: one is the rod cell, which operates under dim light conditions, referred to as scotopic vision; the other light sensitive cell is the cone cell, which gives you sharp vision and color perception.

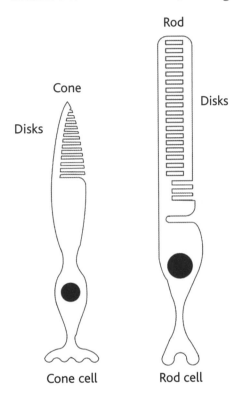

Rod

Cone

Disks

Disks

Disks

Cone cell

Rod cell

Rod cells are the most numerous – about 120 million. They are highly sensitive to low light and motion. Rod cells do not detect color and their visual acuity is about 20/200. For sharp focus and color perception it is the cone cells that are used. These are concentrated in the central fovea located directly behind the iris and the other optical parts of the eye. Cone cell perception is referred to as photopic vision.

There are three types of cone cells, each sensitive to a specific range of light frequencies: the photo-pigments erothyrolabe are sensitive to long-wave red light, chlorolabe is sensitive to mid-range green light and cyanolabe is sensitive to short-wave blue light. The three primary colors red, green and blue enable you to see all the colors in the spectrum. Blending these three basic colors can produce every color imaginable. There are about six million cone cells in each eye with the highest density situated in the central fovea. However, cone cells are present all the way to the periphery of the retina and only about 4 percent of all cone cells are located in the fovea. Interestingly enough, there are no blue sensitive cone cells in the fovea; their peak density lies just outside the central fovea. This accounts for the inability to see very small blue objects when they are centrally fixated.

The rod cells contain the photosensitive pigment rohodosin or visual purple. Named after its appearance, the rod cell consists of about 1,000 tiny disks, with each disk holding about 10,000 molecules of rohodosin. Each molecule is capable of capturing one photon of light. The huge number of rohodosin molecules therefore have tremendous capacity for capturing light. When light falls on a rod cell, the rohodosin becomes bleached. Only one quanta of light is required to bleach a molecule of rohodosin. In fact the scotopic spectral sensitivity of the eye corresponds to the properties of rohodosin.

The macula

The retina has a central area, directly behind the cornea and lens, called the macula. At the center of the macula is the fovea. In this part of the eye vision and color perception are perfectly clear. In the fovea, the photoreceptors have the densest concentration of light sensitive cone cells, approximately 150,000 per square millimeter. These cells are also connected to a very large area of the visual cortex, enabling you to see clearly.

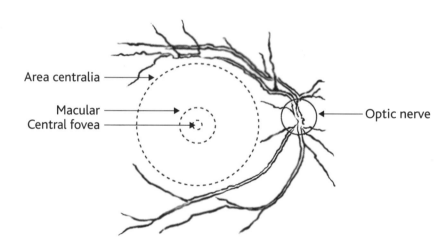

The macula is covered with a yellow pigment consisting of the carotenoids lutein and zeaxanthin. Traditionally it was believed that yellow pigments aided in visual resolution by filtering out the shorter blue light wavelength. Nowadays this filtration effect is considered to be a protection against blue light damage and indirectly a way of squelching free radical oxidation. Incidentally, the distribution of zeaxanthin seems to parallel that of cone cell photoreceptors.

The best dietary sources of carotenoids are dark-green leafy vegetables and yellow and red fruits. Carrots are the best source of beta-carotene and tomatoes supply lycopene. Zeaxanthin is the dominant carotenoid in vegetables such as orange peppers and sweetcorn, while most other vegetables such as cabbage, spinach and watercress are rich in lutein and beta-carotene.

Lutein, taken as a sublingual spray, is one of the most effective ways to stop the progress of macular degeneration, a disease where the integrity of the macula progressively deteriorates.

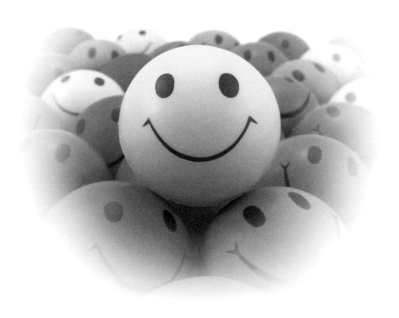

5. Healthy Eyes

Not only are your eyes a mirror of your soul, they are also a reflection of your overall physical health, emotional wellbeing and level of vital energy. Physical exercise is one important factor contributing to your general health. Everyone expects a person to have vibrant wellness if they exercise and are active. Working out and sports are the main activities for keeping fit.

There is a lot to be said for the old adage: "You are what you eat." Nutrition is not really a part of Vision Training, but the information is just too important not to include. I do not believe that I can just take a pill and get clear eyesight. Healthy nutrition is clearly an important aspect of good vision, so it makes sense to create a condition where all the necessary nutrients are available.

What's needed for optimum eye health?

There are two nutrients that are vital for your eyes. The first is vitamin C. The lens, aqueous humor and vitreous humor have about seven times the level of vitamin C than any other part of the body. Vitamin C is an important antioxidant that fights oxidative damage caused by free radicals, spurred on by a photo-reactive process. These start a chain reaction where the end result is the formation of cataracts. Cataracts will cause blindness if not treated. This treatment usually means removing the lens surgically.

The second vital nutrient needed by the eye is vitamin A, which is required for the process of converting light into nerve energy. Vitamin A deficiency is directly related to night blindness. Two other beta-carotene nutrients are important for the proper functioning of the macula – the part of the eye where you have absolute clear vision. Lutein and zeaxanthin supply the yellow coating over the macular region of the eye, which protects the light sensitive cells from damaging blue light.

With the condition macular degeneration – the deterioration of the maculae – the light sensitive cells are damaged and permanent loss of vision is the result. More and more studies link nutrition and poor digestion to the increase in macular degeneration. It used to be a problem afflicting only older people. Unfortunately, younger people are now developing this condition. Currently the most effective way to prevent and deal with macular degeneration is nutritional and most important of all, the sublingual application of lutein.

What can I do to maintain optimum eye health?

I don't believe in mega doses of supplements. My concern is maintaining the body's natural ability to synthesize the nutrients it needs from the food we eat.

Today more people are buying and eating organically grown foods. The beautiful tomatoes you see in the supermarket were most likely plucked green from the plant and artificially ripened during transport to the store. Additionally, the plant was almost certainly enhanced to produce thicker skin and bigger fruits to satisfy your visual expectation of a pleasing tomato – and all this most probably at the expense of nutritional values.

If you have ever eaten tomatoes taken directly from the plant when fully ripened you will know that there is a huge difference. A few years ago I traveled by roads in Mexico that were lined with orange groves. We stopped and bought a sack of tree-ripened fruit. The juice made from these oranges was heavenly and full of vitamin C – grown the natural way. Fruits are generally best in the countries where they grow naturally and can be obtained from local farms.

On the other hand I can't imagine myself eating spinach every day, as one study suggests. I love spinach, but not daily. So the solution is to supplement. I take the word "supplements" quite literally. I take vitamins and minerals as supplements, not as a substitute for food.

Good nutrition is a very confusing topic with trends and opinions shifting every few months. Some purists advocate the advantages of a diet consisting entirely of raw foods. They maintain that heating vegetables to 60° Celsius destroys most of the nutrients. I like salads, but living exclusively on raw food would be a challenge for most people. The middle ground may be the best way to go. So make it a point to include plenty of dark-green and orange vegetables in your salad. Your intake of vegetables is higher if you drink them as juice.

The following is a list of the nutritional elements you need for good eye health. Try to get these vitamins and minerals in your normal diet and supplement as necessary. However, remember that Mother Nature does it best.

Vitamin A

This is vital for natural vision. It is consumed by exposure to heat and glare, flickering fluorescent lights, computer monitors and TV screens. The nicotine in cigarettes and alcohol also burn vitamin A.

Beta-carotene is stored in the liver and converted into vitamin A on demand. It is safer to take beta-carotene since there is no limit to how much you can consume. For vitamin A the limit is no more than 10,000 international units (IU) of vitamin A per day over a long period of time. The recommended supplement dosage is 5,000 to 25,000 IU in a carotene complex.

The best source of beta-carotene is carrots, especially in fresh carrot juice. It is also found in yellow and green fruits and vegetables.

There are two other carotene compounds that are important for the eyes. One is lutein and the other is zeaxanthin. Lutein is the yellow pigment layer that covers the macula. It is thought to protect against the damage of blue light. Zeaxanthin is found mostly in the area of the central fovea where vision is crystal clear.

Lutein comes from vegetables such as cabbage, spinach and watercress. The recommended dosage is 6–20 mg. Zeaxanthin is found in orange peppers, yellow corn and egg yolks. The recommended dosage is 90 mg taken with lutein.

Vitamin B complex

These supplements are best taken together since they must be balanced for the body to be able to absorb them. B complex vitamins are burned up by stress.

Vitamin B^1 (thiamine)

Vitamin B^1 keeps the eye muscles working. It is usually included in breakfast cereals and is found in whole grains, egg yolks, soya milk and milk. The recommended supplement dosage is 10–50 mg.

Vitamin B^2 (riboflavin)

Vitamin B^2 aids with the ability to be comfortable in bright light and appears to play a role in the circulation of nutrients to the lens. Lack of B^2 causes constant eye fatigue, burning eyes and the inability to see during twilight hours. Cataract patients lack vitamin B^2. It is found in almonds, brewer's yeast, milk and soybeans. The recommended supplement dosage is 15–50 mg.

Vitamin B^6 (pyridoxine HCL)

Vitamin B^6 is important for emotional balance. It is found in bananas, brewer's yeast, brown rice, carrots, chicken, eggs, fish and whole grain cereals. The recommended supplement dosage is 50–100 mg. Avoid dosages higher than 300 mg per day.

Vitamin B^{12} (cyanocobalamin)

Below average levels of vitamin B^{12} are apparent in individuals who suffer from cataracts and glaucoma. This vitamin is found in clams, fish, eggs, dairy products and sea vegetables. The recommended supplement dosage is 200–400 mg. Sources of vitamin B are dark-green vegetables, brewer's yeast, eggs, nuts and seeds.

Vitamin C (ascorbic acid)

This is vital for the health of your lenses which contain seven times more vitamin C than any other part of the body. Vitamin C is an important antioxidant – needed to fight oxidation damage by free radicals. Note that smoking diminishes vitamin C levels and is a significant risk factor in developing cataracts. To be fully effective vitamin C supplements must contain bioflavonoids. Bioflavonoids are found in blackcurrants, grapes and cranberries. The recommended supplement dosage is 200–500 mg per day. Natural sources of vitamin C are citrus fruits, such as lemon, lime and orange. It can also be found in melon and tomatoes.

Vitamin D

Vitamin D controls calcium levels and is found in cod liver oil, oily fish and egg yolks. It is usually added to milk.

Vitamin E (α-tocopherol acetate)

This enables the bloodstream to carry necessary oxygen and nutrients to all parts of the body, including the eyes. Vitamin E also appears to be important for maintaining the elasticity of the eye muscles and lens. It is found in wheat germ, almonds and other nuts as well as cold-pressed oils. Avoid the synthetic vitamin E – α-tocopherol. Normally, you will get most of the vitamins you need from the food you eat and from multivitamin supplements.

Calcium

Several studies have found that higher levels of calcium have a positive effect on myopia, detached retina and glaucoma. It appears that calcium dehydrates the fluid within the eyes, thus making the eyeball shorter. Sugar, found in carbonated drinks, appears to be one of the factors that cause myopia. However, when calcium is present, the eyeball reverts back to its normal shape.

Calcium is found in milk, leafy greens and sardines. Calcium should be taken together with magnesium (vital for enzyme activity and energy).

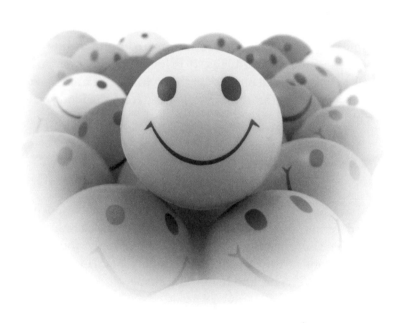

6. Visual Acuity

While the reading 20/20 is commonly held to represent normal vision, most people with good eyesight actually measure better than 20/20. This evaluation represents the upper limit of good vision. Research conducted by Elliot and co-workers (1995) shows a slight decline in visual acuity, from approximately 20/14 at age 25, to just a fraction better than 20/20 at age 75. This is surprising news to most people, since the common belief is that vision starts declining in childhood.

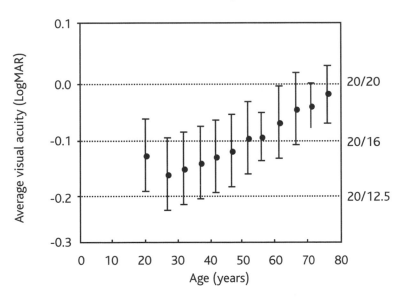

Normal visual acuity with age
after Elliot et al., 1995

Detecting small changes in visual acuity

When you want to detect small changes in vision, credit is given to each letter identified correctly. Research conducted by Baily and associates (1991) has shown that people with normal eyesight identify letters with a 95 percent confidence for changes at ± 5 letters on the eye-chart. If visual acuity is scored row by row, the 95 percent confidence limit for change is determined to be ± 2 rows, because the 95 percent discrepancy lies in the next smallest category, which is ± 1 row. This means that when visual acuity is scored by row, at least two rows of change must occur before a clinician can determine that there has been any real change. Therefore, testing by letter appears to be a more accurate method of measurement.

Decimal acuity

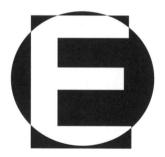

The image of a 20/20 letter E
as relayed to the central fovea
where you have absolutely
clear vision.

With a decimal visual acuity of 1, you can see letters that are 8.7 mm high at a distance of 6 meters. Decimal value decreases with increasing letter size. For visual acuity to be half as good as 1, the letter size would have to be twice as large. For example, for visual acuity to be 0.5, the letter size of the smallest readable letter would be 17.45 mm.

The formula for constructing a decimal acuity chart is as follows. The height of a letter for any given decimal acuity value can be determined by a simple relationship: height of letter = 8.726 mm/decimal acuity. For a letter of a given height, therefore, decimal acuity = 8.726 mm/height of letter. Decimal acuity is used when comparing visual acuity with other variables.

Percentage acuity

Multiplying decimal acuity by 100 results in percentage acuity. Thus the decimal acuity of 1 becomes 100 percent. Percentage acuity can mislead you since it sounds very scary. For example, someone who can only read the top letter "E" of the eye-chart will be told that he or she has only 5 percent vision. Hearing this you think you are going blind!

Letter height	Percentage acuity	Decimal acuity	Metric	English Snellen
4.4 mm	200%	2.0	6/3	20/10
6.5 mm	133%	1.33	6/4.5	20/15
8.7 mm	**100**%	**1.0**	**6/6**	**20/20**
13.1 mm	67%	0.67	6/7.5	20/30
17.5 mm	50%	0.5	6/12	20/40
21.8 mm	40%	0.4	6/15	20/50
43.5 mm	20%	0.2	6/30	20/100
87.3 mm	10%	0.1	6/60	20/200
174.5 mm	5%	0.05	6/120	20/400

Snellen acuity

The common eye-chart is a visual acuity testing system devised by Dutch ophthalmologist Hermann Snellen in 1862, on the basis of what is now known as the Snellen fraction, which is defined as follows:

$$\text{Snellen fraction} = \frac{\text{Testing distance}}{\text{Designation of smallest read line}}$$

Snellen acuity can be stated in either metric or imperial units. The first numbers refer to the testing distance, which is usually 20 feet (6 meters). The second number refers to the distance from which someone with normal eyesight would be able to see this line of letters. So, a reading of 20/40 tells us that a person with normal eyesight could see these letters at 40 feet (12 meters). In other words visual acuity is about half of normal. 20/40 (or 6/12) is also the legal limit for driving without optic correction.

Illumination and contrast

The standard illumination for visual acuity tests is a minimum of 10 foot-lamberts. If you are reading this in daylight the illumination is probably 40 or 50 foot-lamberts in a room with windows. Large windows, on a sunny day, will bring the illumination level up to 100 foot-lamberts. Increasing the illumination does not improve vision, but reducing illumination causes considerable loss of visual acuity. You might have experienced this when trying to read a menu in a dimly lit restaurant.

Contrast is also an important factor. Visual acuity suffers when the contrast goes below 90 percent. One hundred percent contrast is defined as black letters on white background, while 0 percent contrast would be gray letters on an equally gray background – the letters would of course be invisible. Eye-charts for testing contrast are made by altering the gray tones of both background and letters.

Near-vision acuity

This is commonly referred to as reading ability. Near-vision test charts are designed using the same principles that are used for distance vision tests. This text is printed using a 10-point font which makes reading comfortable under most lighting conditions. Normal reading acuity in daylight is 3-point text. The following is printed in a 3-point font:

Doctor: Good morning, Albert ... what seems to be the problem today?

Patient: Well, when I look in the mirror I see sagging jowls, red blotches, thinning hair ... why do I look so awful?

Doctor: I don't know Albert ... but you have excellent eyesight.

Your reading ability is greatly affected by quality of light. Fluorescent light is the least effective while sunlight is the best reading light. Try reading the above story in different light conditions and you will immediately experience the effect.

Presbyopia is a condition affecting your ability to read because your near point of focus has drifted out. Vision Training is highly effective for presbyopia especially if you start exercising your eyes when you become aware of your reading difficulty or before you find that your arm is not long enough to hold a book to read comfortably.

Night vision

At night we rely exclusively on the highly sensitive rod cells. These cells take about 35 minutes to fully adapt to the dark. After about half an hour in darkness your eyes have become 100,000 times more sensitive to light. At night a lighted cigarette can be seen several kilometers away. The military is very aware of this fact, thus the need for total black-out in war situations.

As twilight gradually fades into night, your light sensitive cells also hand over operation from the cone cells used during the day to the rod cells used at night in low light conditions. However, in today's world we seldom experience total darkness. Modern cities have street lights so the total transfer to absolute night vision is seldom completed.

Have you ever had the experience of waking up at night and wondering where the light is coming from? Most likely you realize that the room is illuminated by the digital clock display on your VCR. This is an example of the power of your night vision. It is amazing how much you can actually see with so little light.

Research shows a direct link between night vision and vitamin A. If you have problems driving at night try taking about 5,000–10,000 IU of vitamin A per day.

Contrast

The difference between the intensity of the object you look at and the background is referred to as contrast. Amazingly, our ability to detect contrast does not vary with lighting conditions. Looking at a black print on a white shirt does not vary significantly between indoors in dim light or outdoors in bright sunlight. This consistency in contrast is obtained at the loss of sensitivity. You have probably experienced this whilst reading. The level of black and white contrast is maintained in all lighting conditions. However, it becomes more difficult to read small print in poor light. Your visual system looks for the difference in contrast between the objects you want to see and the background around them. Part of this is also related to vergence. In low light your depth of field – the area where you can see clearly – becomes much smaller. The same phenomenon is well known in photography. With a large aperture opening you get a picture where the background is out of focus. The object therefore stands out against a soft background. Portrait photographers often use this technique to emphasize the face.

To maintain your low light reading ability, try reading small print in dim conditions. I know your mother probably told you not to read in poor light. She was right when it comes to reading a novel with a penlight under your bedcovers. However, it's a good idea to maintain your ability to read small print in varying light conditions. As you begin to experience what small print looks like under different

This is 2% contrast

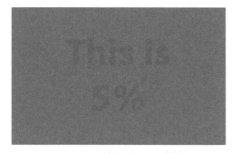

This is 5% contrast

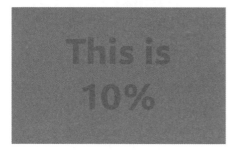

This is 10% contrast

This is 100% Contrast

kinds of light, you should notice how the contrast seems to remain the same, even while your ability to read the text varies.

Loss of contrast after laser surgery

One of the unfortunate consequences of laser surgery is the loss of contrast. After surgery many people find it impossible to distinguish details in an object that is brightly lit from behind. They see something similar to a picture taken of a person against a sunset. Either you can see the sunset and the person is only a shadow, or you can see the person and the sunset is over-exposed. The photographer overcomes this by using artificial light on the person. While driving you often come across situations where your ability to recognize contrast is called for. For example, if you are driving behind a truck with cars coming towards you in the opposite lane, your aptitude with contrast allows you to see both the bicycle between you and the dark outline of the truck ahead. In the pre-surgery consultation the possibility of a significant loss of contrast sensitivity in low light conditions is frequently not mentioned. A little known fact is that many people have to give up driving at night following laser surgery. This is why legislation is under way in the United States and Canada to make it unlawful to drive at night if you have had laser surgery on your eyes.

In Germany, testing for contrast sensitivity is required before you can get a driver's license. Many people who have undergone laser surgery fail this test and consequently cannot get a license.

What is a diopter?

The measurement used to describe lens power is a diopter of the focal length of a lens. If your far point of clear vision is 20 cm, then you will need a 5 diopter lens to correct your vision to normal. The formula is as follows:

$$\frac{1}{\text{Far point of clear vision in cm x 100}} = \text{diopters}$$

The farthest you can see in an absolutely crystal clear manner can easily be converted into diopters using the above formula. Here is an example.

If you can clearly see up to a distance of 20 cm from your eyes, then the above calculation is as follows:

1 over 20 = 0.05. This is multiplied by 100 to equal 5 diopters.

Using the string exercise described on page 83 you can accurately determine your diopter prescription.

Plus and minus lenses

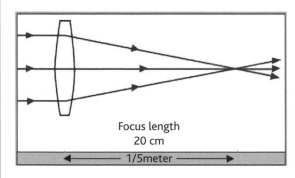

Focus length
20 cm

1/5meter

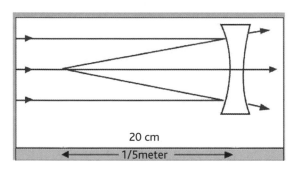

20 cm

1/5meter

Plus lenses are magnifying and bring the near point closer. Reading glasses are plus lenses. These lenses are also used for hyperopia to relieve eyestrain.

A lens with a minus reading of diopters, which is used for correcting myopia, does not have a true focal point because it causes light rays to diverge. The strength in diopters of a minus lens is determined by measuring the distance from that lens to the point where the diverging rays would converge if their path was reversed.

7. Vision: The Mind Side

Vision takes place mostly in the mind. The physical side of seeing is only about 10 percent of what takes place when you are reading this. The optical structures of your eyes – the cornea, lens and the fluid that fills the eye – combine to focus an image on your retina. This is very similar to a camera. The optical part of the camera is your eyes. The film in the camera is your retina.

Conversion of light into nerve energy takes place in the retina. The retina is a very important part of seeing. Color is perceived through three types of photosensitive light cells and, like color film, there are three layers, each sensitive to one of the primary colors. In the retina we have cone cells that are sensitive to red, green and blue light. Yellow is the result of blending red and green; the same subtractive color principle is used in video and television.

The image is now converted into energy flowing through millions of nerve fibers packed together into the optic nerve, which leads to the geniculate body located in the middle of

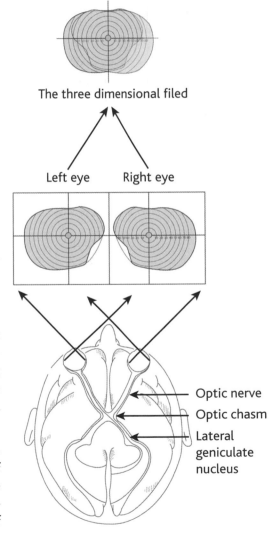

The three dimensional filed

Left eye   Right eye

Optic nerve

Optic chasm

Lateral geniculate nucleus

the brain. Here the nerves branch out. Seeing involves about two thirds of the brain. Many parts of the brain receive input from visual perception. For example, there are parts of the brain that recognize shape, another part perceives color and yet another is in charge of determining where objects are in space. Your peripheral vision is especially sensitive to motion. In prehistoric times, when people lived in the wilderness, it was very important to be aware of danger approaching. Today we use this ability to navigate our way through traffic or down a crowded street.

In Vision Training we involve both the physical part of seeing and the mental and psychological sides. The physical side involves practicing exercises which are designed to relax the eye muscles and affect the shape of the eyeball. This is equivalent to moving the lens back and forth until the image is sharp. With eyesight this is a dynamic process that constantly works to keep objects in focus. Your eyes are far superior to any video camera ever developed. Anyone with normal eyesight can focus on something very close and just an instant later adjust to focus on something far away. Your image is always in focus and crystal clear. A video camera is too slow to make that kind of shift without a cut.

It's a wonderful world out there

All five senses are involved in creating our experience of the world around us. Vision is perhaps the most important of our senses because it serves as the interface between our internal world and the physical reality around us. Your work is likely to involve a significant visual component – seeing what you do, seeing where you drive, seeing a client and so on. This does not mean that you can't function without sight; you can, but it means a significant loss of connection.

For some people, sight is the most important sense. They like to see something before they believe it is possible. In learning, the visually inclined person prefers to see something demonstrated before they can understand and learn. The majority of people in the world belong to that group. Others prefer to hear someone talk about a topic of interest. This is the lecture format used in most of higher education. For these people, the auditory is an important sensory input. Finally, there is the last group of people who need to try something out physically before they really understand it. The kinesthetics are often great craftspeople since they have a feel for the material with which they work. The sense of touch is exceptionally sensitive as well.

Sometimes the senses connect, so that an input of one sense leads to an experience of another. For example, for some people the smell of freshly baked bread triggers memories of childhood. Newly cut grass is another common smell that evokes such recollections. Sometimes a perfume worn by mother or grandmother provides a direct link to memories of days gone by. On other occasions it can be the sense of taste that evokes recollections. Many people tend to order the same dish in a favorite restaurant as the flavor conjures up pleasant scenes from the past.

Certain locations may also bring up memories or feelings. For example, if you go back to the place where you went to school, it is bound to stir up memories. I remember returning to Copenhagen, a city I lived in during the 1960s. Returning 20 years later everything seemed smaller than I remembered. Experiences and states of being can be anchored to specific locations. If you have a negative experience in a certain establishment it is likely that you will choose not to return. If the first impression of a person is less than positive, this tends to color your perception of that individual. Appearances are extremely important. Great chefs spend almost as much time decorating their dishes as they do cooking the food.

Appearance is, of course, the driving force behind fashion. There is no practical reason why we need to change our wardrobe every year. There is no logic that dictates why certain colors are no longer desirable. Fashion goes through cycles. Years go by, and the same patterns and styles come back in some form or other. Shoes cycle through round, square and pointed toe shapes, whilst fabric patterns shift constantly through dots, stripes, flowers and geometrics.

Physical appearance determines how you are perceived. If you are tall, well dressed and young then you are more likely to get the job. The visual aspects of people and objects are of vital importance.

Designers make a healthy living from figuring out what will appeal to your esthetic sense in any given situation. The layout of this book went through several stages of development before we felt that it had the right appeal. The typeface was chosen for its clean appearance and the line spacing to make it easy to read. The illustrations were designed to be visually pleasing. Most attention of all went into the title and cover design. Most likely you bought this book either because of the title or because the cover attracted your attention. After all, vision is the most important sense that we possess.

Where does your attention go?

Your eyesight is directed by your attention. Are you the kind of person who is curious about the world or are you more interested in reading books and minding your own business? If you want to regain your eyesight it is important that you begin to pay attention to what is out there in your environment. Energy follows attention, so if you believe that you can't see, your attention will not reach out very far. The ancient Greeks thought that near-sight was caused by a weak spirit, which did not have the energy to venture out very far. To regain your eyesight you need to consistently direct your attention further and further out into the world. One of the concepts that took me a long time to grasp is the fact that the world only responds to us in relation to how far we throw out our attention. The energy we put out brings back the information we seek. For example, you want to know the time so you look at the clock tower. Your intention shifts out to the clock tower and the energy then comes back to you with the information you seek – the time.

Sensory alignment exercise

The purpose of this exercise is for you to become aware of which sense system is most natural to you – visual, auditory or feeling. This experience will also make you more aware of exactly how your visual system works. Do this exercise without any corrective lenses. It is easier if you do this with a friend to guide you, the explorer, through the experience.

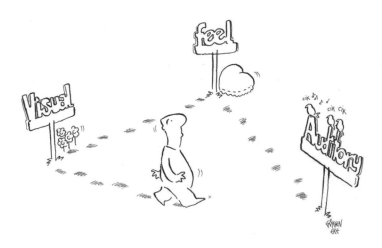

Mark three points on the floor so they are a perfect triangle, with one point for each of the representational systems – visual, auditory and feeling. Make sure the visual has as good a view as possible. If possible, conduct this exercise outdoors.

First, ask the explorer to step into the auditory (the order in which you do the representational systems is not important).

Now begin to become more and more aware of the sounds around you. Become as auditory as possible. You may begin to notice tiny little sounds you were not aware of before. Also notice where in space the sounds come from. Some are very close, like my voice, some are very far off in the distance. When you are ready, begin to move very slowly … very slowly, taking tiny steps and begin to leave the auditory, and very gradually … very gradually move towards the visual. Notice the subtle changes that take place as you gradually move from the auditory to being between the two, and gradually become more and more visual. Now, as you stand there in the visual space, begin to notice the colors, the different shades of colors, and the contrast between light and shadow. Become aware of what's close to you, and now begin to become aware of what's in the middle ground, and what's out there far away in the distance. Let your eyes roam around, jump easily from one object to another. Just enjoy the freedom to move. Let's experiment and see if we can learn something. Find a point or an object that you can see clearly. Fix your eyes there, don't allow them to move. Continue staring at that point without blinking, until you experience a change in what is in front of your eyes. What happens to your visual clarity and your visual field?

[Allow time to experience this.]

Most people find that their visual clarity begins to deteriorate, and their visual field begins to shrink and dim when they stare for a prolonged period of time. Your eyes want to be free and move around. Now, let's do something else that's very interesting. Locate an object that you can see relatively clearly. It can be the same one as before or something different. First, focus on it really hard. Then look at it a second time, but more softly. Notice that the more you focus, the less of everything else you can see. Your entire visual system closes down. Now look at the same object without focusing or staring rigidly and become aware of your breathing. Allow your visual focus to soften and expand … soften and expand, continuing to soften and relax until you can see not only the object but everything around it with the same soft focus. Notice how you can expand this farther and farther until you see everything in your visual field with soft focus … easily and naturally. Everything you see is equally important, and your eyes are in continuous movement. Here and there … out there … over here … moving easily, softly, naturally. You know how you can focus in on one detail and see only that, whilst still seeing the bigger picture? Did you know that you can do both at the same time? Pick an object, then look only at that object. Now soften your focus and bring in the rest of the picture. Keep moving your eyes. They love to roam around, easily, softly, naturally. Now begin to slowly, very slowly, move from the visual towards the feeling. Notice the gradual changes that happen when you begin to move, slowly, noticing all the subtle changes that take place as you move to the halfway point between visual and feeling. Continue to notice and to move towards the feeling. Standing now in the feeling space, begin to feel the ground under your feet. Feel the temperature, begin to sense the flow of air around you. Feel the rhythm of your breathing, easy ... in ... and out. Feel yourself being here right now, completely. Feel the feelings you have and enjoy being fully in touch with yourself and the environment, easily, softly, naturally. When you are ready, begin gradually to move, slowly. Now, move towards the auditory. Begin to sense the subtle changes that happen as you slowly move towards the auditory. What are the changes that let you know that you are beginning to move past the middle point, moving closer and closer to the auditory? Now you are back in the auditory.

Step outside the triangle and talk about your experiences and discoveries. If you like, go around and re-experience each point again. Then ask the following questions:

Show me whereabouts within the triangle you would be when listening to music.

Show me where you would be when watching a movie or visiting an art gallery. Where would you be within the triangle when you are listening to a discussion program on the radio, or when you are listening to a speaker in a seminar? This is an interesting one. Show me where you would be within the triangle when you have a strong intuition that something will turn out a certain way, and you are proved to be right – when you are most tuned in and confident about it. What happens when you change to soft focus?

Finally stand at the center of the triangle having equal access to all senses. What does it feel like?

[Most people feel exceptionally connected and in touch with the world. You have equal access to the three most important input channels.]

Think of three times in the past when you would like to have been this connected. As you cast your mind back, notice how the memory changes now that you have added this powerful connectedness. Go through the memories, one at a time. Select different contexts, for example, one episode may be at work, another may involve the way you interact with people, the third may be a communication with a member of your family. Notice how the memories change.

Now think of three times in the future when you plan to act from this state of connectedness. Again, work with three different contexts. In this way your mind begins to assimilate this resource and make it available to you in your daily life.

Finally make a note of your experience here:

Personalities differ in visual systems

A Chicago-area optometrist who measured the vision of "multiples" as they switched personalities found "remarkable changes." Kenneth Sheppherd (1983: 3) examined three of Bennett Braun's patients in their various personalities. He told *Brain Mind Bulletin* that he found striking changes in such objective measurements as eye pressure and corneal curvature.

One patient needed a correction for near-sightedness nearly four times stronger in one personality than another. When she changed into a 6-year-old, her near-sightedness improved to the point that her original childhood prescription corrected her vision. Her teenage personality required an increase in prescription strength but had better vision than her adult selves.

Far-sightedness, astigmatism and color blindness also changed with a switch of personalities.

8. The Basic Principles of Vision Training

There is the old philosophical division between the objectivist who says, "When I see it I will believe it" and the subjectivist who says, "Believe and you will see." Scientists aim to be totally objective and only believe what they can see and measure with instruments. However, many people feel that a human being is not just an accidental mix of chemicals that happened to fall together. A human being is more than its physical anatomy.

If you adhere rigidly to the objective model then you are limited by the sensitivity of your measuring equipment. Some say that we do not know yet what it is, because we do not have the equipment to measure this phenomenon. Vision is one of the senses that it is difficult to be scientific about. Currently, machines can only give an approximate measurement of the components of your eyesight. Your own perception of vision will always be a subjective one and it will vary from individual to individual. Another example is the perception of color. Each and every one of us has a slightly different perception of color. Science can measure the wavelength of light with precision but your eyes will see it in their own way.

Perceptions can also hold us back. For example, in the 1950s it was considered impossible for people to influence their blood pressure and skin temperature. Then came biofeedback and it became possible to do just that. At one time it was considered impossible to run a mile in less than a minute. For many people it currently seems impossible that one could regain one's eyesight. In fact we can do amazing things. There are many examples of people who have overcome serious illnesses without any medical assistance. Medicine is often powerless in the face of many health problems, yet the human mind has the power to effect very dramatic changes.

A very dramatic demonstration of this is the case of people with multiple personality disorder (MPD). Chicago psychiatrist Bennett Brown conducted an experiment with ten of his MPD patients. He had their eyes measured in three of their personalities. So we have ten people and 30 measurements. To the astonishment of the researchers they noticed objective measurable differences in the curvature of the cornea from one personality to another. Dramatic changes in visual acuity took place within the span of a few minutes as the patients changed from one personality to another. In fact, visual differences are only a minor part of the physical changes an MPD patient can go through when switching personality. Some of them have serious illnesses such as diabetes in one personality and not in others. Some are drug addicts in one personality but in another they can be completely normal individuals without drug dependency.

The multiple personality research is a very dramatic example of how the human body can physically change. Eyesight is really a simple thing to alter compared to serious systemic illnesses that a person with MPD can seemingly put on and take off like a raincoat.

This tells me that eyesight is not a hardware problem, it's a software problem. The mind side of vision is perhaps more important than the physical side. Also, remember that most people are born with natural clear eyesight. Mother Nature has made certain that your most important sense will function perfectly for your entire life.

Your physical vision is what you see when you open your eyes and what happens in between the parts of your eyes that are involved in focusing and the retina. The nerve impulses from the cone cells in the retina develop into what we perceive as vision. This is what we know as the physical part of vision. It relates to what we perceive out in the world.

The larger "software" part of vision happens mainly in the visual cortex located at the back of the brain. Since software can be updated, this is one area where we can effect change in our ability to see.

Beliefs are concepts and ideas that we have taken to represent truth. Our beliefs surround our world like a fence. What lies outside feels to us as if it is not possible or not real. From research we know that the way we define what is believable or real is colored by our own belief structures. Interestingly enough, there are people who have to believe something before it can become real. Others must think of something as real before they can believe it is possible.

If you believe that something is possible then it is clearly much easier to achieve. If you think of something as impossible you are not likely to invest a lot of energy in trying to achieve it. Regaining your eyesight is a lot easier if you believe it to be within the realms of possibility. In fact, one of the main objectives of my two-day workshop is that people leave the session knowing how much influence they have over their eyesight. Of course, knowing what specific exercises you can do is part of that mindset. So let us do a little exercise that will help you achieve more clarity in your vision.

First of all, what is the status of your vision? Do you have near-sight or myopia? Or do you just need reading glasses – the medical term for this is presbyopia. Perhaps you are far-sighted or have astigmatism. Write down what you know about your vision status here:

What do you think caused this? Pause and think about what you believe caused your vision condition to be what it is today. Write it down:

There are many ideas about what causes eyesight to deteriorate. In fact scientists do not yet fully understand what causes myopia, astigmatism and so on. So your ideas are just as good as any others.

For example, do you believe that vision problems are inherited? Many people feel that they have evidence to that effect. There are families where both parents wear glasses and all the children as well. This seems to support the theory that vision problems have a genetic disposition. Yet in other families everyone has good eyesight except one person. This does not seem to support the idea that near-sight is inherited.

Several studies have been undertaken to discover whether myopia is inherited. In the 1950s and 1960s several studies were made with Eskimos in Alaska. The early studies found virtually no myopia among Eskimos of any age. Later studies, made by Francis Young et al. (1969), found about 45 percent myopia in 253 children in one community. However, virtually none of the parents and grandparents of those children had any vision problems. So myopia does not seem to be inherited in the case of Eskimos. In fact, myopia and other vision problems are influenced by a number of genes, so genetic therapy for myopia is not likely for a long time, if ever.

Let me ask you another question. This is a magic question so just let your imagination run free: suppose in your sleep tonight, an angel or a fairy came to you and restored your vision so it was perfect. But since you are asleep you are unaware that this miracle has taken place. When you wake up tomorrow morning, what would be the first thing you would notice as different?

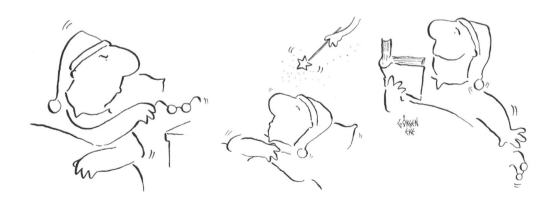

Please write down what it would be like. What would you feel, see and hear?

How would your day be different?

Would the relationship between you and others be different?

Apart from not wearing glasses, what would others notice about you that is different?

What kind of person would you be?

The last question is an important one:

If you'd had perfect vision for the last five or ten years, where would you be in your life and what difference would it have made?

Take the time and really go inside and discover your answers to the above questions. Your mind will begin to focus on your goal of achieving natural clear eyesight. Regaining your eyesight involves not only the physical exercises but also an evolution of your personal identity. You will no longer be the same. You will have changed more than just your visual acuity. Your physical ability to see will have changed as well as your inner vision of yourself, and the world around you will also have changed. Think about it: if you can change your eyesight – what else can you do?

Updating your beliefs about vision

Our beliefs are very powerful. Positive ones can empower us to do amazing things. Limiting beliefs can severely restrict our potential. Beliefs are fascinating just because they are so potent. Beliefs can also represent boundaries around our reality. They filter our experience to fit their purpose. For example, if you believe that you are not a good dancer, this belief may be re-enforced by experiences of less than stellar performances in the real world. Your belief filters, which in this case are limiting, will make you take heed of any circumstances that support this limiting belief about yourself. All the mistakes you make when dancing take on crystal clarity in your mind. Past experiences rise up and add themselves to this witches' brew. The final result is that you feel absolutely terrible and swear that you will never attempt to dance again. So the belief has served its purpose – and you hang up your dancing shoes.

Fortunately beliefs can just as easily reinforce our potential. Beliefs are systemic in nature, so a re-enforcing loop can be either negative – with the situation getting worse and more limiting, or positive – in which case you automatically begin to notice things that support your ability. If you believe that you are a good dancer then you will take notice of all the data that supports your abilities as a dancer, and you will remember how well you dance and how much you have enjoyed dancing in the past.

There are a couple of simple NLP processes you can do that will provide you with some tools to work with your beliefs. In this case the beliefs we are focusing on are the ones that deal with your ability to regain your eyesight. First of all we will explore how you decide exactly what in your life is real and what is not.

Your reality strategy

Knowing the mechanics of how you create the inner code that tells you when something is real for you is of immense value. This is because this pattern can be used to reinforce the things that you want to experience strongly in your reality. Here is a way to check out the way you interpret your world.

1. Think about what you had for breakfast this morning. How do you experience this memory? Do you see the breakfast table in front of you? Notice whether you see this through your own eyes (associated), as if you are part of the scene, or do you see yourself as outside the picture looking in? Is the image in color or black and white? Also notice whereabouts in space this image is located in relation to yourself. Are there any sounds? Does the memory also include the sense of taste? Are emotions involved? Notice all the sensory qualities that make up your experience. Write down the sensory qualities of how you experienced your breakfast.

2. Now change one element of your experience. For example, if you had cereal, change that into something else you might have chosen. Suppose you'd had toast instead, now how do you experience the scenario? Go through the same modalities you checked out before and notice if there are any changes. There are likely to be one or two significant differences. In some cases these will be obvious. For instance, the picture may now have become black and white, whereas it was in full color during the real experience. For other people the differences may be much more subtle. The position in space where the image resides is often of great significance. If the picture moved out by say 10 cm, that could be the difference in your world between something that seems real and something that is imaginary. Write down the way you experienced the imaginary scenario here:

3. Compare the two experiences and check each sensory modality for image quality, color, position in space and so on. What about sounds and feelings? Find the one possible element that makes the difference between the two experiences.

4. The final step is to check whether you have found the key difference. Do this by thinking about something in your life which you would like to have accomplished but you have not yet brought to fruition. For example, it could be something you would like to own but is not yet in your grasp. It could also be a skill you would like to possess. Modify the way you think about it and reproduce the configuration your mind uses when it thinks about something that is real. The result should be that you begin to have doubts as to whether the thing you desire is actually real or not. If you get to this stage – well done, you have found your reality strategy. Write it down here:

Knowing your personal reality strategy is an important element to achieve if you want to take advantage of the powerful technique of mental rehearsal. It can help you discover the difference between a so-so experience and something that is truly exceptional.

Your belief strategy

How do you decide that something is believable? What does it take to get you to believe that something is true? Are you 100 percent convinced to the point of knowing something to be an absolute fact? Your beliefs are a continuum between something being completely unbelievable to believing with great certainty. Obviously knowing just how much you believe something can be immensely valuable to you. Here is how you can work out your own belief strategy.

1. In your mind's eye, visualize something that you know for certain – something there is absolutely no doubt about. For example, do you believe that the sun will rise tomorrow and there will be another day? Do you believe that the earth

is round? There might be people who have doubts about these things, but you get the idea.

Again, make an internal inventory of how you experience this. The image quality and position of the image are often key elements in a belief strategy. Check image qualities such as colors, motion and distance. In some cases a belief can also be experienced as a feeling in a specific part of your body. For instance, you might experience certainty as a particular feeling just below the ribs. Otherwise it might be a sense of feeling firmly grounded. Think about how you experience something that is absolutely certain to you. Note it down here:

2. Next think about something about which there is a degree of uncertainty – something that you believe might possibly happen, but you don't know for sure. For instance, do you believe that the U.S. currency will go up in relation to the Euro? Do you believe that you will get a salary increase this year?

Now check out how you experience this. Notice the differences and similarities to the feeling of absolute certainty in the last exercise. Does the position of the image change? Is the feeling the same? Note it here:

3. Finally, think about something you absolutely do not believe in – something you think is totally false. For example, do you believe in beating children to make them learn a lesson? (I hope not!) When you think of something along these lines, notice how you experience it. Whereabouts in space is the image? Is the feeling different from before? Write down the details here:

You probably already have an idea about how your beliefs are coded. It is likely that there is one modality that changes in proportion to how certain you are about something. This is your belief strategy. Use a few words to write it down here:

4. Now we come to the final discovery. For some people something has to be perceived as real before they can believe it. Others start with the beliefs and things start to become real afterwards. Check for yourself how your system works. Think of something you would like to have as a reality in your life. First clothe it in your reality strategy modalities and then move it into the spatial position that you now know means that you believe something with absolute certainty. Notice how this feels. Does it make the experience more powerful?

Then reverse the sequence and check whether it is more powerful for you if you believe something with absolute certainty before you move the experience into your mind's configuration for something that is real.

Now you have one of the most important tools for getting your mind to work for you and help change limiting beliefs. This is equivalent to a master's degree in visualization.

The belief change cycle

We are constantly changing and updating our beliefs. For example, as a 4-year-old child you believed that it was dangerous to cross the street without an adult holding your hand. At one point you probably also believed in Santa Claus – I still do!

NLP developer Robert Dilts found that beliefs go through several stages as they update and change. The first stage of a belief change is a feeling of uncertainty. You don't believe your belief quite as much anymore. The belief has moved down the certainty scale. If you are open to doubt, then you are open to belief. The new belief seems more attractive. It is moving up the certainty scale. At one point you can simply let go of the old belief. Dilts suggests that you place it in your "museum of old beliefs." This is an ingenious way of keeping the old belief in such a way that it no longer influences you. It is something you used to believe that is no longer relevant. Finally, the new belief becomes a certainty. Take your old beliefs about your ability to regain your eyesight through these stages and empower yourself. Remember – seeing is believing.

Old belief
↓
Open to believe
↓
Museum of old beliefs
↓
Wanting to believe
↓
New belief

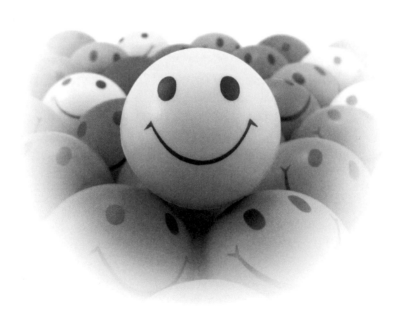

9. Exercise Your Ability to See

Apart from believing it is possible to change ones eyesight we also need to recognize the importance of physical and mental exercise. When your glasses do most of the focusing for you, your eye muscles begin to lose their tone due to lack of use. It is common knowledge that regular exercise leads to better health. In this book I have outlined a number of specific exercises for particular vision problems. In general there are just two or three exercises you need to do in order to experience an improvement. Depending on how severe your myopia is you may need to go through several sets of exercises before you begin to regain your natural eyesight.

The visual system is closely connected with memory. This makes practical sense since such a huge amount of information can be stored visually. You may experience this in words or concepts. Your memory is employed in figuring out the pattern that the individual letters make in the formation of a word. You have probably had the experience of looking at something but not being quite sure at first what it was. Your internal visual database was flipping through several possibilities until you finally realized that you were looking at a part of a car, for example. Your mind had successfully connected the visual shape, color and so on to that object. This is experienced as a knowing. The same is taking place at a much faster pace as you are reading these words. Your eyes are taking in the patterns that are formed by the letters, whilst your inner database comes up with the meanings of the words and phrases. The internal visual experience is as important as the external. In fact most of your visual experience actually happens in the brain.

You also have inner vision. I find it very interesting to note that many people with myopia also tend to have smaller internal images in their mind's eye. It seems that the minus lens reduces the size of the world to fit their internal perception – a smaller image. Often eyesight improves if we take steps to adjust this imbalance.

How to discover your internal vision

The properties of your inner vision have great influence on how you perceive the world. For example, if everything you saw was in black and white, what would that mean in terms of how you experience your reality? How would it feel? Let's play around a little with this.

Recall a memory of something very pleasant. Look at this memory as if through your own eyes and as if you are present experiencing the experience right now, so that you are associated into the experience. Feel the feelings. Now, change it around so that you are looking from the outside in at yourself in that situation having that experience. What has happened to the feelings? Did you become less involved and more detached from the feelings?

In the field of neuro-linguistic programming we call these shifts submodalities. Any change you make to the quality of any aspect of a submodality has an impact on how you perceive the world. For example, things that are close-up and large usually have more impact than things that are far away and small. Colorful images are more attractive than black and white. Images that move are more interesting than still pictures and so on.

Find your dominant eye

You can work out whether the left or right eye is the dominant one, but this can change over time, so this is only valid at the time of testing.

1. Look at something that you can easily remember – perhaps a flag or a letter on the eye-chart. Place both hands together and create a small gap which you can peer through. Look at the object you have chosen to work with. Look with both eyes at the object through the opening between your hands. Slowly begin to move your hands towards your eyes and keep looking through the gap with both eyes. When your hands touch your face you will find that you will be looking through them with your dominant eye. This may come as a surprise to you. Many people discover that their dominant eye is actually the one they had considered to be their bad eye. Make a note of which eye was the dominant one.

2. Look at the object, and then open and close your eyes a few times until you get a good image of it in your memory.

3. Close your eyes and look at the memory image. Notice which eye you are using.

4. Now look at the memory image with the other eye. Is there a difference in the quality of the image?

5. Take the image that appears to be the clearest and use your imagination to make the other image the same. In some cases the images may be of different sizes or in different locations. If this is the case, then mentally move the images so they inhabit the same space. Make it so the image that appears to be the clearest is on top as if you had two slides of the same image and had laid one on top of the other, as if making a sandwich.

6. When you have a nice sharp internal image then slowly open your eyes and look at the original physical image. Notice if there is any difference between the inner image and the physical image. If so, then make the image appear to be the same size internally as well as externally. The object is to find the configuration that produces the clearest image.

I have noticed that many people with myopia discover that their internal images are smaller than the related physical images. This is interesting because minus lenses, used to correct myopia, are actually shrinking the images so they become smaller. The reverse is also the case. Many people with presbyopia discover that their inner pictures appear to be larger than the physical images – plus lenses magnify the world.

Balancing your imaginary and physical vision

The purpose of this exercise is to discover exactly how your brain processes visual information. For instance, you may be amazed to find that you actually see better if you imagine your eyes to be at the back of your head, or perhaps if you visualize your imaginary eyes to be 5 cm out in front of your physical eyes. In my case I get better contrast if I imagine my eyes are at the back of my head. It is like turning up the contrast on the TV. When I imagine my eyes to be out in front of my actual eyes then I get one more line on the eye-chart, or 5 percent better visual acuity. This exercise requires a good level of dexterity with the imagination so it may not be suitable for everyone. In any case I suggest you have fun experimenting and finding out what works for you.

This exercise is done with your eyes open. We want you to find out the optimum configuration that will enable your eyes to get better.

1. Look at an eye-chart or something which is detailed enough for you to find out if your vision is improving. Imagine that your eyes are mounted on wheels so

that they can roll to the back of your head. This may be easier to do if you move your hands back at the same rate as your imaginary eyes move. Notice what happens. Does your vision appear to get better?

2. Next move your imaginary image to the middle of your head. What happens to your vision?

3. Move your eyes back to their normal position.

4. What happens if you move your imaginary eyes 5 cm out in front of your physical eyes? Does your vision get better? Move your eyes back to their normal position.

5. This time move your imaginary eyes 10 cm further apart. What happens to your vision? This is useful for trainers because you can suddenly see the whole room. What happens to your vision?

Move your eyes back to their normal position.

6. Next, discover what happens if you move your imaginary eyes upwards so that you see the world from above. One of my participants in Brussels suddenly realized that she had been reading through the eyes of her childhood. Moving her eyes upwards enabled her to immediately begin reading through her adult eyes.

7. Finally, move your eyes downwards. Does this make your vision better? One participant in Berlin discovered that her sight became much better with the imaginary eyes located somewhere near the outer corners of her lips.

This exercise takes advantage of the fact that vision is mostly a mind activity. By giving your brain new and unusual instructions, you discover new and possibly better ways of using your eyes. Since you are only moving your imaginary eyes nobody will notice that you briefly moved your eyes to the back of your head to read a street sign.

Are you avoiding what you don't want to see?

The relationship between mind and body is becoming increasingly accepted. For this reason, Vision Training incorporates exercises that are designed to shift long-standing psychological and mental patterns. Playing about with what works will eventually become the natural way of being. Psychological and emotional aspects of our reality have enormous influence on eyesight. In 1962 Charles R. Kelly researched this issue and found that what we should not, must not or would rather not see can be blurred or blanked out by the mind. In my work with vision problems over the last ten years a pattern has emerged. A typical belief is that if people believe there is something in their immediate experience that they do not like they are helpless to do anything about the situation. If this dynamic goes on for a long time the mind will simply dim one's vision so the problem is no longer visible.

A typical example illustrating this dynamic is a lawyer friend of mine. She attended a Vision Training workshop given by Janet Goodrich years before I started my project of regaining my eyesight. We shared information about techniques that worked. However, her vision did not improve significantly. I suggested that we explore this one-on-one.

During this exploration of what might be the root cause she told me that during her childhood her father had a relationship with a cousin. She felt bad about this and did not want to see it. Over the years she had talked about how lawyers in the office had affairs with each other and with clients. My friend was practicing family law where infidelity is a common reason for seeing a lawyer. I pointed out to her that as far as her subconscious was concerned the pattern that caused her eyesight to deteriorate in the first place was still going on in her immediate environment.

My friend had a very stable relationship with her husband, so I suggested to her that she need not take responsibility for other people's conduct. Apparently her subconscious mind agreed because a few days later she called me and very excitedly told me about the amazing progress she had made in just a few days.

Without rediscovering whatever decision you made in the past that keeps your eyesight below par, you will see flashes of clarity, but they probably will not last. One woman in Ireland had studied the Bates Method for three years. She came to my class because she had never been able to go past flashes of clear vision. When I told her there probably was something in her past that needed to be processed before her subconscious mind could permit clear eyesight, she said, "Yes, I think I know what it is."

At the subconscious level there is no time and space – only now. So if something happened to you as an 8-year-old, that inner child is still with you. The emotional imprint is still active even if you have consciously forgotten all about the event. In my workshop I do a short regression exercise which creates a context in which your subconscious can help you discover what might be the inner reasons for keeping your vision dimmed.

People usually discover innocent associations made by the mind of a child. For example, one man told me that he realized he had made a connection between wearing glasses and wisdom. As an 11-year-old he wanted very much to be like his dad – who wore glasses. A woman told me that her twin sister was fitted with glasses, so she faked the test. She wanted to be like her sister.

One exceptional case that dramatically illustrates this dynamic involved a 7-year-old girl in London whose vision went from normal to -4 diopters in just ten days. After some investigation her mother discovered that this little girl had been bullied in school and had concluded that absolutely nothing could be done to improve her situation. She could not stop the bullying herself and did not believe that her parents or teachers could help her either. Consequently, her mind dimmed her vision.

Psychologists researching attention have discovered that vision can collapse by as much as 60 percent towards the near point when people were asked to solve math problems that were very difficult or impossible for them to work out. This may be one of the reasons why so many children start to have vision problems.

10. Getting Energy to Flow

In China the system of acupuncture is a major part of the country's medicine. The aim of the Chinese approach is to achieve a balance between the yin and yang energies. One of the basic models in Chinese medicine and acupuncture is the concept of the five elements. According to this model the healing energies flow from water to wood, to fire to earth, to metal and back to water. This journey also describes the seasons of the year. Each element is associated with one of the major organ systems of the body.

The water element is considered to be a winter energy and is associated with the bladder on the yang side and the kidney on the yin side. The wood element is the energy of spring and is associated with the gallbladder, which is yang. The yin side of wood energy is the liver. The fire element is summer energy. On the yang side it is associated with the small intestine and the triple warmer. On the yin side it is associated with the heart and circulation. The earth element is Indian summer and equinox. The spleen is on the yin side and the stomach is on the yang side. Finally, the metal element is autumn energy, which is associated with the lungs on the yin side and with the large intestine on the yang side. This completes the circle.

Across the circle there are lines of energy that enhance or balance these elements. The five-element model enables the Chinese medicine practitioner to know whereabouts in the system he should intervene in order to achieve optimum balance and health. Around the eyes and the head there are many acupuncture points which can be targeted to direct energy. As mentioned above, we want to have a free flow of energy through the eyes and head. If the energy flow is blocked, the organs, in this case the eyes, are depleted in energy and will function less efficiently.

To get the energy flowing we can use pressure or massage – acupressure – rather than needles. With acupressure we use the fingers and two basic movements. The first is press and release, and the second is small circular movements in counter-clockwise movements to release energy and clockwise movements to energize. It is good practice to do three counter-clockwise movements first to cleanse and then clockwise movements to energize.

The Five Elements

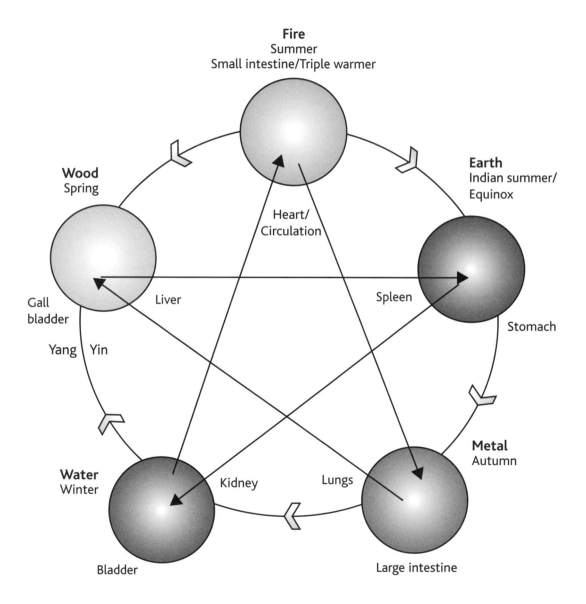

Chinese acupressure for your eyes

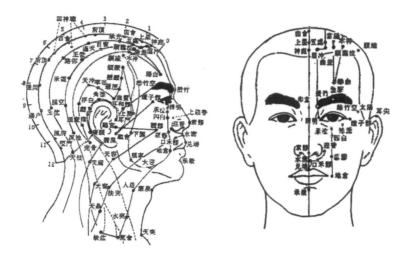

There are ten steps in this exercise. The purpose is to get the energy flowing through your eyes and head. You may notice that some of the points feel slightly tender. This indicates that energy is not flowing very freely at that particular point. The massage movement will start things moving again and you will feel a wonderful freshness and openness after this exercise.

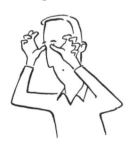

1. The first point – bladder meridian B2, which improves all eye problems – is located at the root of the nose and up under the eyebrow. Place the tip of your thumb as close as possible to the inner corner of the eye and press upwards. You will sense a tender spot right where the point is located. Rotate three times from right to left (counter-clockwise) to cleanse and then left to right (clockwise) to energize. You could also just press and release several times.

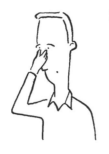

2. The second point – bladder meridian B1, which also improves all eye problems – is located on each side of the root of the nose, right where the petals of your glasses normally rest. Use your thumb and index finger and grip the root of your nose. Make three circular movements right to left (counter-clockwise) and then left to right (clockwise) movements to energize. Alternatively, you can just press and release.

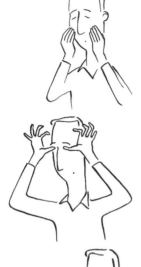

3. The third point – stomach meridian ST3, which improves cataract and swelling under the eyes – is located on the cheekbone at the same level as your nostrils, about one and one half fingers outwards. Use three fingers and you are sure to touch this point. Do three circular movements right to left (counter-clockwise) and then left to right (clockwise) movements to energize. Alternatively, you can also just press and release.

4. The fourth step involves several acupuncture points along the bone over your eyes (gallbladder GB2 and triple warmer). Begin where we found the first point, then move out in small steps across the bone to the outer corner of the eye.

5. Next comes the bone under the eye. At the inner corner of the eye we have the first point of the bladder meridian. Directly underneath the center of the eyeball we have the first point of the stomach meridian, ST1, which relieves red eyes, night-blindness, too many tears and also near-sight. The easiest way to do this is to use four fingers and press down and release on the edge of the bone. Sometimes you will feel a wonderful coolness flowing down over your eyes, indicating the flow of energy.

6. The next step is the gallbladder GL1 point, located at the outer corners of the eye. Massage with three circular movements right to left (counter-clockwise). Then energize with left to right movements (clockwise).

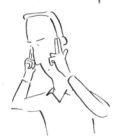

7. Next move to the hairline to the TW22 point on the triple warmer. Massage with three circular movements right to left (counter-clockwise). Then energize with left to right (clockwise) movements.

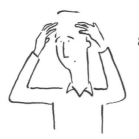

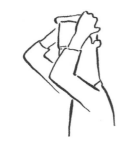

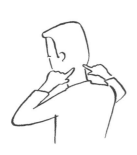

8. Move a bit further back, placing your fingertips on an imaginary vertical line moving up from the ears. Massage the four points beneath your fingertips. This is the gallbladder meridian. Massage with three circular movements right to left (counter-clockwise). Then energize with left to right clockwise movements.

9. This movement is often referred to as the "tiger climbing the mountain." Open and close your fingers as if they were claws, just as you do when you are washing your hair. Start from the hairline and move up and back towards the center of the head, using one long smooth movement. You can use the soft part of your fingers (if you have long finger nails) or you can use your nails. Put some pressure on to get the energy flowing. With this one move you touch more than 15 acupuncture points on each side of your head.

10. The final point is located at the back of the head just where your neck muscles are attached to the skull. You will find some indentations on each side of the head – this is where the 20 gallbladder points are located. Massage with three circular movements, right to left (counter-clockwise). Then energize with left to right movements.

This energy moving exercise can be used as many times as you like. It is especially useful to do when you feel that your head is getting a bit woolly as the exercise gets the energy moving around your eyes and head. As you can see, there are many beneficial acupuncture points involved in this simple exercise. Also I suspect that it might encourage hair growth. It is an exercise you can do with any vision problem and feel the benefits from it.

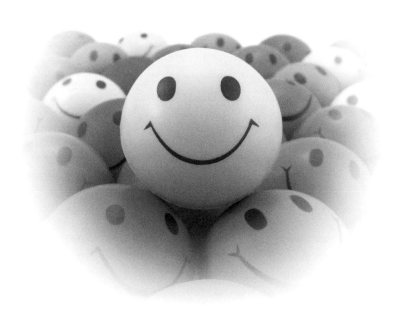

11. Check Your Eyesight

Relax and see

Natural clear vision is effortless – you simply open your eyes and see. Problems arise when we begin to force our visual system. As we grow up, and especially when we start going to school, we learn to repress our internal signals. If a 4-year-old child feels sleepy she will rub her eyes – it is a signal that she needs rest. Somewhere along the way we learn to stifle this natural urge and tension builds up in the visual system as we begin to use more and more force to accomplish visual tasks. Or we simply continue reading way past the time when the eyes need a break.

Near-point tension develops when we attempt to hold the focusing system steady on the book we are reading for too long. Research shows that even short periods of stress require several hours of recovery. This may explain the relationship between academic achievement and vision. Sadly a doctorate is often accompanied by myopia.

Our eyes were designed to be used in a constantly changing variety of circumstances, not just for reading or using the computer. People working in occupations where their vision is used over fluctuating distances generally have much better eyesight. For example, how many cowboys do you see with glasses? Members of tribal or native societies seldom have any visual problems. They live in close harmony with nature and their lifestyle naturally maintains their good vision. I know of an anthropologist who went to Peru for two years to live with the peasants there. Before she made the trip she always wore glasses. However, when she returned from her voyage her eyesight had once again become normal. None of the peasants in Peru wore glasses, so after a while the anthropologist started doing without her glasses and eventually her eyes reverted back to the way that nature had intended her eyes to be.

How to test your distance vision

First of all you need to know the status of your vision. If you have been to an optometrist recently then you will have an idea of your current visual prescription. If you suspect that your vision is beginning to change, then take this opportunity to test your own vision using the enclosed eye-chart.

The eye-chart on pages 84 and 85 are designed for viewing at 3 meters, so find a place where there is good daylight and measure out the 3 meters on the ground. Place sticky labels on the floor to mark the spots that indicate 1, 2 and 3 meters away from the chart.

Test both eyes

Now stand on the 3 meter marker and observe the chart with both eyes. Which line can you see? Note the lowest line on the chart where you can make out the letters. They do not have to be crystal clear, just good enough for you to be able to identify the letters.

Write the result down here:

          20/   6/

Test your left eye

Cover your right eye with your hand. What is the lowest line where you can identify the letters? Note it down here:

          20/   6/

Test your right eye

Cover your left eye with your hand. What is the lowest line where you can identify the letters? Note it here:

          20/   6/

If you can't see the first letter of the eye-chart from a 3 meter distance then you have more than 5 diopters of myopia and you need to do the vision check with the string which is explained on page 86.

In summary

If you can see the 20/25 line then you have only slight myopia and may only need to do eye exercises for a few days to correct to 20/20.

See page 109.

If you can see up to the 20/30 line then there might be a bigger problem but it is still manageable by doing the eye-chart exercise on page 110.

If you can see the 20/40 line then you can still drive legally without glasses, but it is time to take the Vision Training exercises seriously.

See pages 113–118.

How to check if your myopia is more than 4 diopters

Visual acuity is directly related to the furthest point that you can see clearly. There is a linear relationship between the distance to your far point in centimeters and the power in diopters needed to correct your vision.

You will need a piece of string about 1.5 meters long, a bookmark shaped piece of paper/card with text printed on it (about 16-point font) and two differently colored ink markers.

1. Tie a knot at each end of the string so you have something to hold on to. Tie the string to a chair or ask someone to help you with the measurement.

2. Hold the knot on the string under the middle of your eye on the top of the cheek so that you are looking down the length of the string. Close the other eye.

3. Hold the bookmark against the far end of the piece of string, and bring it inwards to identify the point where you start to be able to see the top line of

Improve Your Eyesight Naturally

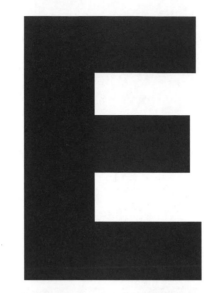

Metric system		Snellen
6/133	**E**	20/400
6/120	**KR**	20/200
6/48	**LVD**	20/160
6/3.5	**ZSHC**	20/125

Metric system   **Snellen**

6/24	# CHGKRN	20/80
6/21	## DCNRSPKE	20/70
6/18	## HONGSDCV	20/60
6/15	OKHGDTNVRCS	20/50
6/12	YOUCANDRIVENOW	20/40
6/7.5	BDCLKZVHSROA	20/30
6/6.75	HKGBCANOMPVESR	20/25
6/6	YOUHAVEPERFECTEYESIGHT	20/20
6/4.6V	THISISEVENBETTERYOUHAVEMAGICEYES	30/16

Designed for viewing at 3 meters.
Letter size and distance is important for accurate measurement. Please download this
chart from www.vision-training.com/en/Download/Download.html

text. Find the point where it becomes crystal clear. Mark this point with one of the marker pens. This is your far point for that eye.

4. Next, bring the bookmark in further to find the closest point at which you can see the top line of the bookmark with absolute clarity. This is your near point of clear vision.

5. Repeat the whole process with the other eye, using the other colored marker.

6. You now have the far point and the near point of absolutely clear vision in both eyes.

7. Place the two knots together and pull the string straight. You can now see if there is a difference between the near point between your eyes' near and far points.

Calculate your eye power in diopters

Measure the distance in centimeters from the knot to the far point. If there is a difference then measure the far point for both eyes. The formula for calculating this is as follows:

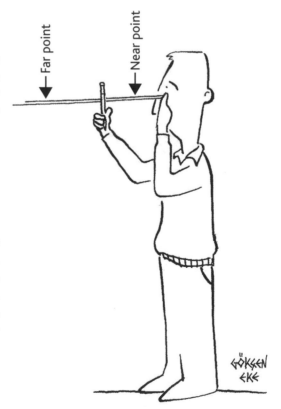

$$\frac{1}{\text{Far point in cm} \times 100} = \text{diopter}$$

For example, if your far point in one eye measured 20 cm from the knot, the diopters will be 20 over 1, which equals 0.05. Now multiply by 100, which is 5 diopters. With this method you can accurately determine the visual acuity of your eyes.

The significance of the near point

Normally the near point should be about 15 cm from the knot. If your near point is further out then you may be presbyopic (in need of reading glasses). In any case you need to do exercises that will bring your near point back to or very close to 15 cm.

Presbyopia occurs when you have difficulty reading but still have excellent distance vision. If your near point of clear vision is more than 25 cm out then you should start doing the presbyopia exercises on pages 136–139.

Also check if you have astigmatism using the chart on page 92.

Now that you have measured your visual acuity go to the pages that describe the exercises you need to do to regain your eyesight.

On the following page there is a near vision test which you can use to determine your near vision acuity.

Near vision test

Observe the test chart in good daylight using the normal reading distance (about 35 cm). Notice which line you can read comfortably. This will indicate your reading acuity. If you can read the bottom paragraph then you have perfect near vision.

Distance in cm	Diopters
100	1.00
80.0	1.25
65.0	1.50
57.0	1.75
50.0	2.00
44.5	2.25
40.0	2.50
36.5	2.75
33,0	3.00
30.5	3.25
28.5	3.50
27.0	3.75
25.0	4.00
23.5	4.25
22.0	4.50
21.0	4.75
20.0	5.00
19.0	5.25
18.0	5.50
18.5	5.75
16.5	6.00
15.0	6.50
14.0	7.00
13.0	7.50
12.5	8.00
11.5	8.50
11.0	9.00
10.5	9.50
10.0	10.00

20/100	# Sight is mind and eye co-ordination.
20/90	It is more mental than physical. The eye sees, but the mind must interpret and evaluate what is seen.
20/80	There are five basic components of mental sight: curiosity, contrast, comparison, memory and judgment.
20/70	Curiosity means intelligent visual searching (i.e., looking around you as if you could see everything with perfect clarity).
20/60	Counting objects and colors is the best way to achieve curiosity.
20/50	Contrast is the gradation of difference between foreground and background.
20/40	For instance, the print on this chart will appear blacker if you close your eyes for a moment and clearly imagine a sheet of clean, white paper before you open your eyes again.
20/30	Comparison is the evaluation of similarity and difference. A capital "H" and a capital "N" both have two parallel sides; but the "H" has a horizontal bar, while the "N" has a diagonal line.
20/25	Memory is the sum total of our learned and our remembered experiences.
20/20	Judgment is the summation, the end result, the interpretation or evaluation of what the eye sees.
20/16	Always use daylight whenever possible. When reading or working at night be sure to have adequate light consisting of the full spectrum of colors. The best combination of working light is a halogen pin light with a dimmer switch illuminating your working area. On the left side there should be an incandescent light and possibly fluorescent light fixtures in the ceiling. Fluorescent light alone is the worst working light as far as your eyesight is concerned.

If your reading vision is less than 20/25 at your normal reading distance, then you need to do the presbyopia exercises described on pages 136–139.

The basic idea is that you need to have extra capacity so when your eyes get tired you will still be able to read at a comfortable reading distance.

Look at this chart in good daylight using the normal reading distance (about 35 cm). Notice which lines you can read comfortably. This will indicate your reading acuity.

Note that lighting influences your ability to read. Daylight is the best quality light you can read by, whilst fluorescent light tubes produce the worst kind of light for reading or working.

12. Astigmatism

In the normal eye all light rays are seen to bend in the same direction. In astigmatism the light rays vary from plane to plane. Typically the cornea has the greatest refractive power at the vertical meridian, the 12 o'clock–6 o'clock line of the watch dial. This is known as "against-the-rule" astigmatism or direct astigmatism. Research indicates that this is by far the most common type of astigmatism and is found in around 88 percent of all cases.

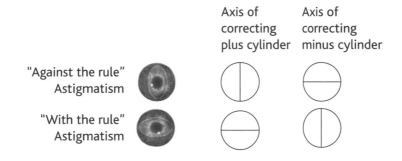

The less common "with-the-rule" astigmatism occurs when the refractive power of the cornea is greater along the horizontal meridian, or the 9 o'clock–3 o'clock line on the watch. About 5 percent of all cases are with-the-rule astigmatism. However, it is possible to have astigmatism at any point of the compass and to have horizontal as well as vertical astigmatism at the same time. You can have astigmatism in only one or both eyes and/or you can have astigmatism at different angles in each eye.

The conventional explanation is that the fault is inherent in the eyeball – either in the cornea or the entire eyeball – which is presumed to be congenitally distorted. Ophthalmologists generally define astigmatism as caused by the toroidal anterior corneal surface.

In other words, astigmatism is an irregularity in the curvature of the cornea caused by tension and pressure on the eyeball. In rare instances, astigmatism can form in the lens or in the retina.

Optically, astigmatism is corrected by the combination of spherical and cylindrical lens elements that form a complex curved shape, somewhat like the sections of a football. To make this work the optometrist needs to define the axis of the refractive error – two lines at right angles to each other – which indicate the greatest and least degrees of the error. He must also ensure that the lens is worn in exactly the right position.

Contrary to traditional belief, astigmatism is very fluid and is usually easy to correct – relaxation is the key.

Astigmatism is one of the vision problems that responds beautifully to Vision Training. I have seen mild astigmatism (less than 1 diopter) vanish after just a few exercises. Some time ago I gave an introductory talk at a conference held at Regent's College in London. In the audience there was a woman who remarked that some of the lines on the eye-chart seemed to be darker than others (this is a sign of astigmatism – see the astigmatic mirror on page 92).

After guiding the group through the Tibetan wheel exercise (see below) I showed the woman the astigmatic mirror once again. She cried out, "It's the same, it's the same." Everybody assumed that she was talking about the astigmatism; in fact she was talking about the lines on the astigmatic mirror. Suddenly everyone realized that the astigmatism had gone after just one exercise. Astigmatism does not always go that fast. However, most people will notice that a change has taken place.

In most cases astigmatism will disappear after exercising for just a few days. With more severe cases it may be necessary to do the Tibetan wheel exercise for a few weeks before the eyes return to normal.

Vision Training principles for astigmatism

- Exercise the exterior eye muscles at a gradual pace, so they become more flexible.
- Get feedback in the form of an astigmatism chart. It is important that you know how you are progressing.

There is growing evidence that the development of astigmatism is formed by environmental influences as well as the personal visual habits that you have adopted. The rigidity of the cornea, which may vary individually from person to person, also plays a role. The flexible corneal tissue reflects the stress patterns influencing the eye. This is similar to putting up a tent. If you don't maintain equal tension in the wires your tent will tilt in the direction of the wire you have tightened the most.

In Vision Training we adopt the presupposition that astigmatism is mainly caused by tension carried in the rectus muscles located around the eye. Consequently, the best strategies for correcting astigmatism involve exercises designed to loosen or adjust the tension held in those muscles. Many of the body's muscles are kept on a continuum between being totally relaxed to very tense. Your neck muscles are a good example of this – you have probably experienced having really tense neck muscles at some point in your life. During the day you maintain a delicate balance between tension and relaxation in order to keep your head movements flexible. You are ready to move in any direction the very instant your attention is drawn to something in your environment.

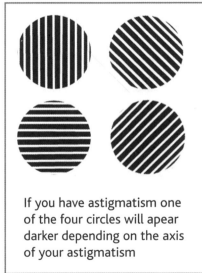

If you have astigmatism one of the four circles will apear darker depending on the axis of your astigmatism

Astigmatism can develop when the upper and lower rectus muscles (the four muscles that control the eye's movements from left to right and up and down) are too tense. This results in an excessive up and down pull which causes the cornea to curve more along the vertical meridian (the 12 o'clock–6 o'clock line). It flattens slightly along the sides, producing typical with-the-rule astigmatism. Since astigmatism is caused by tension in the muscles around the eyes, the best way to correct it is to release the excess tension. In the following exercise we will explore a couple of ways you can quickly identify which of your muscles are tense, and then begin to relax them.

First, look at the astigmatic mirror or the circles above and identify your current state. Try looking at the chart from several distances. For some people there is astigmatism at certain distances only. Find out if your astigmatism is more pronounced close to or far away. If so, this will be valuable information later on when you want to check your progress.

Note that the astigmatic mirror will only be accurate within the field of your clear vision. Outside the range of your natural vision the chart is not reliable. However, as your vision continues to improve, the chart will stay accurate. As you exercise, check the astigmatic mirror from time to time to monitor your progress. You will notice that the darker lines begin to even out or the lines will begin to appear to be of the same length all around.

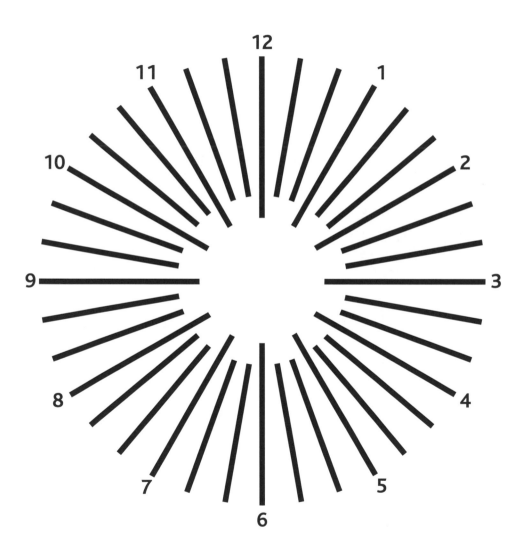

Exercise to loosen the eye muscles

This exercise is designed to gently loosen the muscles of your eyes before attempting more strenuous exercises. The objective is to induce flexibility in the muscles. If you find this exercise is painful then go slowly. Don't attempt the Tibetan wheel exercise before you can do this exercise very comfortably.

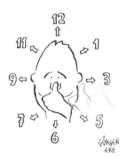

1. Place your thumbnail straight ahead in front of your eyes. Your thumb should be less than the width of your hand from your face. Some may not see the thumbnail clearly. This is all right since we only want to exercise the muscles.

2. Now, very slowly, move your thumbnail straight up. Keep your head still and follow the thumb up as far as you can see. Then, very slowly, move your thumb straight down. Continue to move your thumbnail to the various angles shown on the drawing.

3. When you have done one round of this, relax your arm and eyes for a moment. When you are ready, do the same exercise again, but this time synchronize your movements with your breathing. As you are moving your thumb up, inhale, and as you are moving your finger down towards the center exhale as slowly as you possibly can. Notice how your entire body begins to relax, including your eyes.

4. Do this exercise with synchronized breathing once in a clockwise direction and once in a counter-clockwise direction.

Did you find that moving towards some of the angles was more difficult than others? This is an indication that your rectus muscles are less flexible at those angles. Check your progress on the astigmatism chart on page 92.

Do this exercise three times a day with a few hours of rest in between. It is a kind of aerobics for the eyes. You want to just touch the tension and then relax. Doing this repeatedly over a period of time will loosen up and greatly reduce any tension you have in your eye muscles and, as a result, your corneas will begin to revert to their natural shape.

Tibetan wheel exercise

This exercise will stretch your eye muscles much more due to the sharp angle between the Tibetan wheel chart and your eyes. By moving your eyes in various steep angles around the dial you begin to stretch your eye muscles and as a result they begin to recover their normal flexibility and your corneas will revert to their original shape, thus restoring clear natural vision.

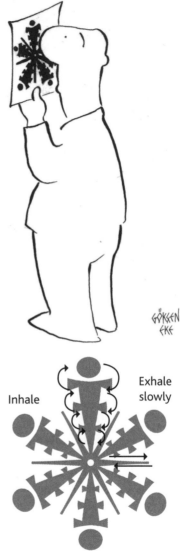

1. Place the Tibetan eye-chart about 2.5 cm from your nose with the tip of your nose at the white circle in the center. You may not be able to see the chart sharply; the purpose is to exercise your eye muscles.

2. As you inhale let your eyes jump up from step to step until you can see the ball. Then let your eyes jump down the steps at the same rate as you exhale, as slowly as possible. Let your entire body relax.

3. Let your eyes follow the smooth spikes. Inhale as you go out and slowly exhale as you come back towards the center.

4. Continue around the chart, first in a clockwise direction, then in a counter-clockwise direction.

5. Do this exercise three times a day with a few hours of rest in between. Check your progress by looking at the astigmatism chart on page 92.

How to move your eyes

Some people like to play slow relaxing music as they do this exercise. The rhythm of the music will enhance the calming effect. As mentioned earlier, astigmatism is normally quite easy to eliminate through the exercises outlined above. In many cases just a few days of regular exercise is enough to restore normal clear eyesight. You will know you have achieved this when you can move your eyes

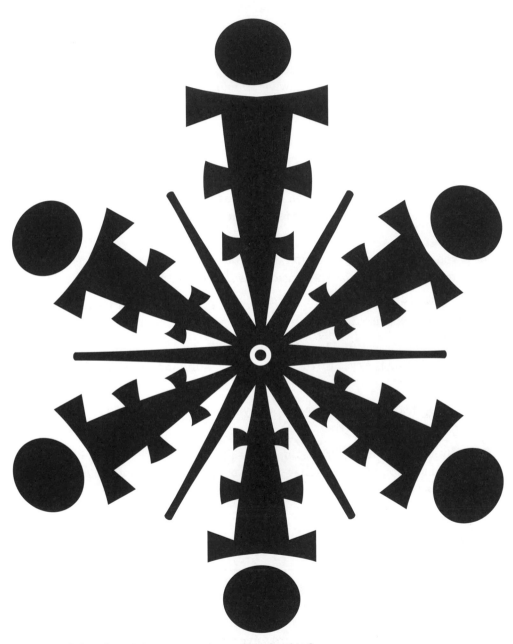

The size of this chart is important please download it from
www.vision-training.com/en/Download/Download.html

easily in all directions and see the astigmatism chart on page 92 clearly without distortion. Remember to look at the chart from several distances and particularly where you noticed any distortion prior to your exercise program.

The exercises are safe as long as you do not over-exert your eye muscles. Take it easy and allow your muscles to regain their natural flexibility over a few days or weeks. What's worth doing is worth doing well. Should your astigmatism return you now know what to do.

Exercise without the chart

If you have astigmatism in one eye or the axis of the astigmatism is different in each eye, you can do this exercise to release the specific muscle group that holds the tension.

By now you have ascertained at what angle your muscles are most tense. For example, you may have found that the tension lies along the 2 o'clock–7 o'clock axis.

1. Hold a finger or a pen about 3 cm from your eyes and move it back and forth along the axis three times. Each time go as far as the eyes will go.

2. Now, close your eyes and imagine yourself doing the same thing, except that you are moving the eyes further in each direction. Imagine yourself doing this three times.

3. Next, do the exercise again with your eyes open. You will notice that you can move your eye a bit further.

4. Finally, do the exercise for the opposite axis as well (the 11 o'clock–5 o'clock axis). This is done to ensure that you are not just shifting the astigmatism from one axis to another.

Some objective proof

Astigmatism is identified on topographical images of the eye as a "bowtie" pattern (see the following picture). A topographical image can be compared to the lines on a map which show the contours of a landscape. The images you see on this page are taken one day apart and offer very impressive evidence of how effective eye exercises are for astigmatism.

October 30, 1999

October 31, 1999

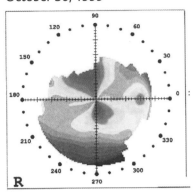

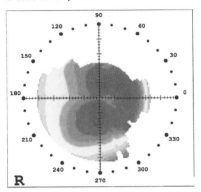

[OD (Right) Data]
<Ref. Data>
S: +1.00 C: -0.5 A: 83

[OD (Right) Data]
<Ref. Data>
S: +0.75 C: A:

The image on the left shows half a diopter of astigmatism (C: -0.5). Note the typical bowtie pattern which indicates the axis of astigmatism, in this case 83° (A: 83).

The image on the right shows the same eye the next day after Vision Training exercises. You can see that the red color has spread, indicating that the eyes have returned to normal and no longer measure any astigmatism. The eyes have also regained +0.25 diopter of hyperopia. This is objective proof that Vision Training is effective for astigmatism.

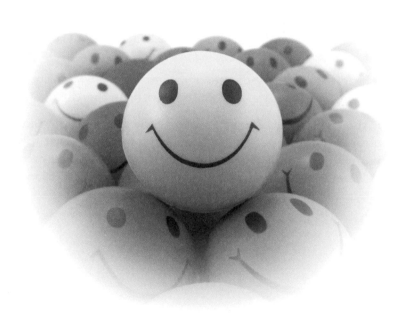

13. Myopia

Near-sight or myopia is the most common vision problem and will touch the lives of almost half the population at some time or another.

When you experience the first signs of myopia, you can still see what's going on in your immediate environment quite clearly. It is only objects in the distance that appear blurred. Myopia usually starts during the school years when you begin to realize that you have trouble seeing what is written on the board. At first it is easy to cope with but it soon becomes more of a problem. You get your eyes tested and then usually get fitted with glasses. However, as soon as you begin to wear glasses you find that the myopia only tends to progress and worsen. You will then need a stronger prescription in order to see comfortably. Soon you find that you are wearing the glasses the whole time, when the truth is that you could see perfectly well without them.

What causes myopia?

The loss of distance vision has been acknowledged since ancient times. The Greek concept of myopia was that too little "spirit of vision" poured out of the brain and hence the vision was too feeble to extend to a distant object. However, not much attention was paid to vision problems until the mid-nineteenth century. Interestingly enough, during the first half of the century the use of glasses was discouraged. They were thought to aggravate the existing problem and be harmful.

During the 1860s, German ophthalmologist Herman Chon observed that myopia increased as children progressed through school. In 1867 Dr. Chon published a study of the eyes of 10,000 children attending the schools of Breslau. He arrived at what seemed a reasonable conclusion: namely, that use (and, in particular, abuse) of the eyes was what caused myopia. Chon's theory dominated for the next 50 years and a crusade began for better standards of visual hygiene in schools throughout Germany.

The Dutch ophthalmologist Franciscus Cornelius Donders believed that myopia occurred as a result of prolonged tension on the eyes during close work and the elongation of the eyeball. In *On the Anomalies of Accommodation and Refraction of the Eye*, he writes:

> How then is this prolongation explained? There are three factors to be taken into consideration: 1) Pressure of the muscles on the eyeball in strong convergence of the visual axes; 2) Increased pressure of the fluids, resulting from the accommodation of blood in the eyes in the stopping position; 3) Congestive processes in the fondus oculi, leading to softening, even in the normal eye, but still more under the increased pressure of the fluids of the eye, giving rise to extension of the membranes. This increased pressure causes the extension to occur principally at the posterior pole, and is explained by the want of support from the muscles of the eye at that part. (1864: 343)

Accommodation

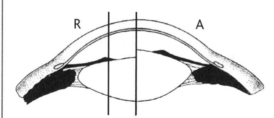

Accommodation is a theory first suggested by German scientist Hermann von Helmholtz in 1863. It refers to the refractive state of the eye due to change in the curvature of the lens in order to focus a sharp image on the retina.

When the ciliary muscle, which is located around the lens, contracts, the tension decreases to allow the lens to bulge out and become thicker. The thicker lens is said to have *accommodated*. The right-hand image (A) shows the lens accommodated.

On the other hand when the ciliary muscle relaxes, the lens is pulled out and it becomes thinner. This is referred to as the *un-accommodated* state.

Accommodative amplitude refers to the distance from the eye to the point of the first slight sustained blur or far point, converted into diopters. This is the *clinical amplitude*.

Until the invention of equipment that could accurately measure the size of the eyeballs in a living human being, it was believed that the ciliary muscle got weaker and could no longer focus the lens. This theory is still offered as the explanation for myopia by many eye-care professionals. Ultrasound scans have shown objectively that with a high degree of myopia there is an elongation of the eyeball. What causes that elongation is a matter of opinion. Some researchers thought that the problem was increased pressure in the eye. For example Kelly et al. (1975) refer to myopia as "juvenile expansive glaucoma." However, the pressure theory is unlikely, since both coughing and an increase in body temperature cause an increase in intraocular pressure.

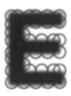 ## When vision blurs

When the optic elements of the eye focus the image on the retina you have sharp vision. If the image is out of focus the image on the retina will form *blur circles*.

Just as in the case of the aperture in a camera, the depth of field varies in the eye according to the diameter of the pupil. The relative size of the blur circle increases in proportion to the distance of the optical image from the retina. In myopia, the optical image is located in front of the retina and consequently you perceive an out-of-focus image.

Blur circles differ according to the shape of the object in view. For example, a line will look like a series of small blur circles (object points) one above the other. On the other hand, a two-dimensional image, such as an eye-chart, is formed by lots of blur circles following the shape of the letter you are looking at.

Pinhole glasses take advantage of this phenomenon. The many tiny holes decrease the blur circles with the result that you perceive a clearer image. Pinhole glasses generally give you an idea of what your vision would be like if fully corrected.

In a study published in 1969, Coleman et al. demonstrated changes in the axial length of the eye with accommodation. Young (1801) and Bell (1827) both suggest that increased vitreous pressure, resulting from sustained accommodation during prolonged near vision, plays an important role in axial elongation and the development of myopia. This seems to correlate with the experience of computer users and others involved in near work.

Peter Greene (1980) evaluated the stress experienced on the eyes based on engineering principles. He examined the stress forces on the sclera by accommodation, convergence, vitreous pressure and the external eye muscles. Greene concluded that the mechanical effects of convergence completely dominate those created by accommodation, even though both occur simultaneously when the eyes focus on a very close target. His calculations show that the total stress experienced by the posterior sclera is the sum of the stress induced by intraocular pressure and by the oblique muscles. He found that the region between the two oblique muscle attachments is subject to a tensile strength higher than those at any other location of the eyeball. This theory, therefore, could account for the axial lengthening of the eyeball that occurs in high myopia.

New York ophthalmologist William H. Bates (1915, 1918), after four years of research into the accommodation and focusing of the eye, came to the conclusion that the oblique muscles are the major factor in the focusing of the eyes. He believed that the ciliary muscle and the lens were only of minor importance.

Contact lenses

Many people use contact lenses every day for years. There have been great advances in the construction of lenses and new materials have been developed.

However, when wearing anything in the eyes you are increasing the friction between the lens material and the protective protein layer, which starts to wear off. This protein is important because it forms the first line of defense against organisms which can cause potentially blinding corneal ulcers. When you wear contact lenses some of this protective protein rub offs. This is unavoidable. The older the lenses are the more friction and consequent damage they cause. For example, a torn or chipped contact lens creates an abrasive edge that can scratch the cornea.

Contact lenses also permit less oxygen to get to the cornea. In other words the cornea is suffocating. Even well-maintained contact lenses continue to accommodate protein. As you clean the lenses the cleaning fluid breaks down this protein. However, some of the modified protein still remains on the lens. You begin to react to this "foreign protein" in much the same way as you would to a bee sting. The immune response causes small bumps to form on the underside of your eyelids. These bumps known as papillary hypertrophy increase sensitivity to contact lens wear.

Think of contact lenses only as a temporary solution while you train your eyes. Use them as a training device.

Bates and others have noted that some people who have had their lenses surgically removed can still see better than 20/40. In other words, a person with no lenses in his eyes could still drive a car legally. The legal limit for driving is 20/40 visual acuity.

There was a woman who attended my vision training workshop in Vienna who'd had an operation to remove her lenses as a child. In those days it was not possible to insert artificial lenses, so she had lived most of her life without any lenses. After the Vision Training workshop she found that she could read text printed in an 8-point font, and she could see the 20/30 line on the eye-chart from 3 meters. She was an inspiration to all of us and a reminder of how fixed our perceptions can be: no lens, no eyesight. Scientific facts tell us that the lens constitutes a maximum of 10 percent of the refractive power of the eye.

Theories about what causes myopia abound and there are many proposals for classifying the problem. Let's make it simple and think of the causes of myopia as functional myopia and structural myopia.

Functional myopia occurs when you are using your eyes too much for near work, such as working at a computer all day. This near work requires you to do a lot of reading while keeping your focus more or less within half a meter. It goes back to Herman Chon's (1866) observation that over-use of the eyes for near work is the main cause of myopia. Essentially, you are gradually training your eyes to focus only on near objects and neglecting to exercise your distance vision. For example, animals raised in a close environment develop myopia. There is solid scientific evidence that environment has an influence on eyesight.

William H. Bates (1915) suggested that myopia occurs because of mental strain. This actually makes sense when you think about how vision problems vary in different parts of the world. In areas where there is not such a great emphasis on reading and book learning, vision problems are virtually non-existent. Garner et al. (1988) examined 977 Melanesian schoolchildren between the ages of 6 and 17 on the Pacific Island nation of Vanuatu. In two examinations conducted in 1985 and 1986 they found myopia greater than 0.25 diopters in only 1.3 percent (1985) and 2.9 percent (1986) of the children. In other words they all had good eyesight.

In contrast Lam and Goh (1991) found that the prevalence of myopia in Hong Kong schoolchildren was almost 30 percent at age 6 to 7 years, just under 60 percent at age 10 years and 74 percent at age 16 to 17 years.

In Hong Kong, Singapore and Taiwan children spend many hours every day doing school work which involves a lot of reading and near work.

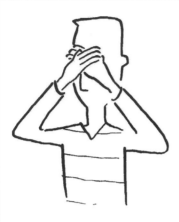

Palming

Palming is the hallmark of the Bates Method. Dr. Bates realized that vision problems were mainly caused by mental strain, so he was always searching for ways to relax the eyes.

The effect of palming your eyes is that your vision becomes clearer. Sometimes you may see flashes of clear eyesight when you remove your hands. At other times it could take a few moments before the vision clears.

To palm, start by rubbing your hands together, as you would do on a cold day. This action warms your hands.

Then place the palms over your closed eyes in such a way that all light is blocked. It is easier if you cross the fingers over your forehead.

You enhance the relaxation response if you exhale as slowly as possible and imagine blackness inside your eyes. When you are completely relaxed you perceive a deep blackness – like black velvet.

If you see gray shadows or sparks of light, it indicates that you hold tension in your visual system.

Reading the Bates literature you get the impression that palming for extended periods is the best practice. I recommend that you palm for a maximum of one minute at a time and do it often, so your eyes remain as relaxed as possible.

The pressure of life on the pacific island of Vanuatu is very different from the pressure exerted on Chinese students. Firstly, learning to read and write the Chinese character script takes many hours of concentrated effort. Secondly, there is extensive preparation for the very strict examinations that are the foundation of the Taiwanese school system. By contrast, the children on Vanuatu are using their eyes to look at things at all distances, and are therefore more likely to be able to maintain their natural clear eyesight. Compare this to the children in Taiwan, who start the task of learning to read and write at 4 or 5 years of age. Writing 100 perfectly formed characters, all exactly the same size, requires a lot of concentration and predominantly focuses their eyes on their books. The children end up over-using their eyes at the near focus, which causes mental strain and subsequently the onset of myopia.

In all reported studies of myopia, none of them have found the condition at birth or present at a very early age in more than 1 to 2 percent of the population. In fact, 98 percent of all 5 and 6-year-olds have good eyesight. It is a fact that most of us start out with natural clear eyesight but by the time a child reaches the age of 15, the prevalence of myopia is something like 20 to 25 percent.

What happens during the first ten years of school? This period is very formative in physical and emotional as well as mental aspects. Psychological studies on the area of attention have found that if a student is requested to solve difficult or challenging mental problems, the focusing of the eyes tends to collapse towards the near point by as much as 60 percent. Imagine a 9-year-old in a math class struggling with fractions. All his friends understand them, but he just can't get his mind to comprehend what they are all about. He tries to concentrate harder and probably begins to turn inward towards his feelings. Difficulties in school often come up as one of the root causes for vision problems in children.

The *structural myopia* theory suggests that genetic factors cause the eyeball to elongate and myopia to develop. Goldschmidt (1968) provides an extensive review of the literature on genetics in myopia. He concludes that genetic factors are important, but there are several types of myopia with different genetic patterns. Other researchers have found no basis for the genetic myopia theory.

As you know, the conventional approach is to fit anyone who is myopic with corrective minus lenses. This will appear to give you good vision as long as you wear the lenses. The lenses themselves do absolutely nothing to improve the condition; on the contrary, the experience most people have is that they will require stronger and stronger lenses. Unfortunately, the myopia becomes progressively worse.

Other approaches involve refractive surgery using laser beams to essentially carve the corrective lens into the surface of your cornea. Like all surgery this involves some risks especially when you consider that the cornea is only half a millimeter thick – roughly three pages of this book. Obviously there is not much room for error and the result is irreversible.

Myopia can vary from very mild (less than 2 diopters) to quite severe (more than 4 diopters). So we have to look at Vision Training strategies for each of three main degrees of severity. Obviously the lower the diopter required to correct the vision, the easier it is to train the eyes to function normally.

Colored eye-charts

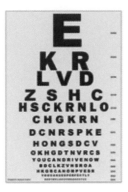

Colors are focused at different points along the optic axis. For example, the color blue has a shorter focal length than red. Using an eye-chart that has a red background on one side and a green one on the other means that people with myopia will notice that the letters on the red side appear sharper. Research indicates that the total chromatic aberration interval (from red more distinct to green more distinct) is from 0.50 to 0.75 diopters.

We use different colored eye-charts to make it easier to see progress by working with a color contrast that suits the eyes.

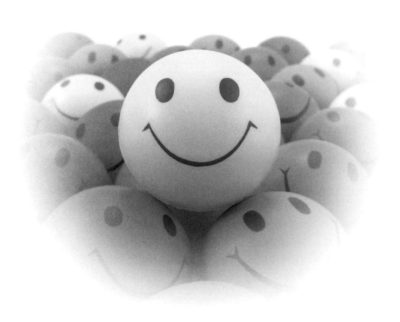

14. Recovering Myopia of Less Than 2 Diopters

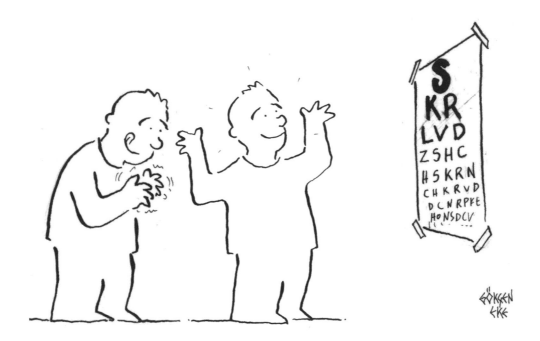

This is mild myopia that only interferes with detailed vision at a distance. You can recover from this fairly quickly by doing eye exercises and following this advice:

● Wear lenses only when absolutely necessary. You do not need glasses for reading and deskwork. Give your eyes a chance to adjust.

● Work with the eye-chart to see lower and lower lines, finally moving down to see the bottom line clearly.

- Develop the habit of moving your eyes from near to far objects.
- Sharpen your vision by swinging (see below).

How to practice with the eye-chart

The eye-chart (Snellen card) serves as a feedback device for you to monitor your progress. The objective is to be able to see as many lines down the chart as possible. Place the chart in a spot where there is good daylight. Measure out the exact distance of 3 meters and place markers at 1 meter intervals. Here are Dr. Bates' recommendations for practicing with the eye-chart.

1. Place the eye-chart on a wall in good daylight.

2. Place yourself 3 meters from the chart and read as far as you can without effort. Alongside each line there are small letters indicating distance. Along the big letter "E" the figure is 20/400, so this size letter can be read at a distance of 400 feet (130 meters) if the vision is normal. The second to last line on the eye-chart can be read from a distance of 3 meters.

3. Now, let's say you can read as far down as the fifth line. You will notice that the last letter on that line is an "N." Now palm your eyes and remember the "N." This mental picture will help you to see the letter directly below, which is a "D." Continue this process down the chart.

4. If you stare at the last letter on the line you will notice that all the letters on that line will blur. It is beneficial to close your eyes briefly and shift to look at the first letter. Alternate blinking and shifting your attention from the first letter to the last letter. You will find you can read all the letters on that line by closing your eyes briefly for each letter.

The eye-chart exercise is especially useful when you have just 1 or 2 diopters of correction. With more than 5 diopters you can't see the first letter of the chart.

The best distance to train with the eye-chart is the place where you can work with the lower half of the chart. As you get to see more and more lines you move away from the chart. Finally you will be able to see the 20/20 line from a distance of 3 meters.

Swinging

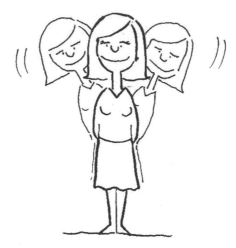

This is another exercise developed by Dr. Bates to relax the eyes and develop sharpness. There are several ways of doing the swing.

The simple sway

1. Stand with your feet slightly apart so you are firmly grounded. Place your awareness on the eye-chart and find a line where you can distinguish the letters but cannot see them clearly.

2. Begin to sway your body from side to side. Allow your eyes to sweep across the line back and forth three or four times. Close your eyes and stop swaying.

3. When you feel centered, open your eyes and find one letter on the line. Look at the top part of the letter and then look at the bottom part of the letter. Allow an opening to take place. You will notice a sharpening of the letters and possibly the entire line.

The long swing

With the long swing you are turning your body at the waist, moving in a 180° sweep. You allow your eyes to slowly trace objects in the environment. In the beginning work rather slowly. Speed is not important – simply practice in the way that is most relaxing. Do the long swing at different distances in space. You will notice that things begin to become clearer.

The eye swing

This swing is performed only with the eyes. Look at a word or short sentence and sweep across from beginning to end several times. Briefly close your eyes and then look back at the word. You will discover that it is now clear.

Centuries ago the Japanese Samurai discovered that during archery training the warriors who visually followed the path of the arrow to their target experienced an improvement in their visual skills. Even those who had normal eyesight found a significant improvement in their ability to see. The Japanese master might say to his students, "Look at the tree, then look at a single branch, then look at a single leaf, then look at the veins in the leaf, and finally look at the tip of one leaf." In essence, this variation of focus provides a key to natural clear eyesight.

15. Recovering Myopia from between 2 to 3 Diopters

This is the mid-range of myopia. At 2 diopters you have clear vision out to about 50 cm. You will be comfortable reading and doing close work without glasses. For computer work you might need to pull the monitor a bit closer to you so the screen falls within your visual range.

At 3 diopters your vision extends out to only about 35 cm. This is fine for reading but for working with a computer it might be too close for comfort. Your prime objective will be to regain 1 or 2 diopters so that you can work comfortably.

There a number of exercises for correcting between 2 and 3 diopters of myopia:

1. Use the string exercise to move your far point of clear vision out. You only have about 15 cm to go before you get to 2 diopters.

2. Use the chart-shifting exercise to practice shifting from near focus to far focus. Start with the larger text and then go to the smaller text block when you have gained some experience.

3. When you get closer to 2 diopters begin to do some exercises with the eye-chart. You will probably find that you are somewhere on the lower half of the chart.

4. Practice the swinging exercises described above and do the domino exercise described on page 116.

Chart-shifting exercise

The purpose of this exercise is to train the ability to shift focus between near and far. It develops accurate saccadic fixation and spatial location by shifting from a hand-held chart to a wall-mounted chart.

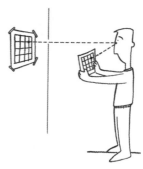

1. Place yourself just far enough away from the chart so that it is a bit of a challenge to see clearly.

2. Holding a small eye-chart in your hands, read three letters aloud in your mind. Then blink as you shift and read the next three letters from the wall chart, and say them out loud.

3. You have the option to alter the way you read the letters. For example, you can start from left to right as in normal reading. As an alternative, you can also read the letters going up and down in columns. Or you can start from the end and go back towards the beginning. Finally, you can select three letters at random and find the next three letters on either the wall chart or the hand-held chart. The ultimate challenge would be to spell names by reading each letter alternately from the wall chart and the hand-held chart. The important thing is to keep your mind interested and have fun with the exercise.

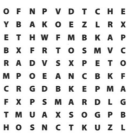

```
O F N P V D T C H E
Y B A K O E Z L R X
E T H W F M B K A P
B X F R T O S M V C
R A D V S X P E T O
M P O E A N C B K F
C R G D B K E P M A
F X P S M A R D L G
T M U A X S O G P B
H O S N C T K U Z L
```

4. To enhance the focusing powers of your eyes move both towards and away from the wall chart while attempting to see the letters clearly at the maximum distance possible. Do the same thing with the chart you are holding in your hands. To improve near-sight move the charts further away. For far-sight and presbyopia move the charts closer and closer.

5. Do this exercise for a few minutes, then rest your eyes by palming. The aim is to accomplish the shifting process as quickly and accurately as possible. Exercise for a maximum of 5 minutes each time. Keep in mind, however, that it is beneficial to do this exercise frequently.

The same action described in this exercise can also be done in other environments at school or at work. Switching from one focus to another, combined with a slight challenge in terms of moving the blur zone further away, is a very useful exercise particularly when you are in the mid-range of myopia. You can also combine this

O F N P V D T C H E

Y B A K O E Z L R X

E T H W F M B K A P

B X F R T O S M V C

R A D V S X P E T O

M P O E A N C B K F

C R G D B K E P M A

F X P S M A R D L G

T M U A X S O G P B

H O S N C T K U Z L

You can download this chart from
www.vision-training.com/en/Download/Download.html

exercise with tromboning (moving closer and further away – see page 164) while you are attempting to keep the image sharp.

The domino exercise

This is the "swinging" exercise introduced by Aldous Huxley in his book, *The Art of Seeing* (1943). The purpose of this exercise is to improve the sharpness of the eyesight by getting the eyes to learn to relax. The marked contrast between the white dots and the black domino makes it easy to get good results. I have found this exercise to be very useful for extending clear vision for those with less than 2 or 3 diopters of short sight.

1. Start by palming your eyes for 1 minute.

2. Find the distance from the illustration where you can see the domino pattern clearly. Step a little further back, so that the dominoes become soft. Not blurry, just soft.

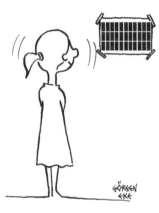

3. While swinging your head slowly from side to side, let your eyes run over the first line of dominoes. You are not looking at any particular domino. Just let your eyes glide over them. Notice the white margin, the edges of each domino and the white dots.

4. Close your eyes and keep moving your head as if you were looking at the first row of dominoes. Exhale as slowly as possible as you do this.

5. Open your eyes and look at the dominoes as they swing by. Notice what happens. Move further and further away as your vision improves.

6. Close your eyes once more and sweep by the first row of dominoes in your mind.

7. Open your eyes and sweep across the second row of dominoes. Alternate between swinging across the page with eyes open and closed, as if you were reading the lines all the way to the bottom of the chart.

Look at the dominoes as if they were columns. Allow your mind to become involved by adding up the dots and calling out the total as you read each domino. For example, the first domino has only three dots. The second has two and six dots, so say

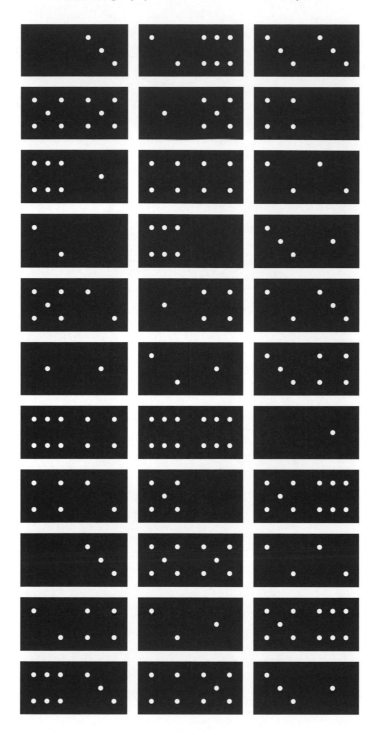

eight, and so on. You can also add up the entire line of dominoes. Play around with this exercise three or four times a day and you will find that your vision will become perfect in no time at all.

16. Recovering More Than 4 Diopters of Myopia

With 4 diopters of myopia your vision extends out to only about 25 cm, which is too close for reading or working. With higher degrees of myopia you have even less visual range and you may have found in the past that you need to wear glasses the whole time in order to function.

The basic principles for regaining eyesight of more than 4 diopters of myopia are:

● Always wear lenses that are about 1 diopter under-corrected. This will give your eyes room to improve.

● Make sure that you have enough energy in your eyes for them to work comfortably. Low energy limits your progress.

● Work with the string exercise (below) to first equalize your eyes so both left and right eye have the same near point and far point. Then begin to move the far point further out.

● Decrease your lens prescription as you progress.

If your myopia registers anywhere from 4 to 14 diopters you are looking at several months to several years of Vision Training. Your eyeballs have to make some major changes before you have clear natural vision again. The first step is to wear reduced prescription lenses. If you continue to wear the full prescription, the glasses or contact lenses will do most of the focusing for you. Your eye muscles are used to doing very little and over time become lax and lose their tone.

Wearing glasses causes your eyes to adjust to the lens prescription of the glasses themselves. A friend of mine wanted to avoid serving in the military, so he borrowed the spectacles of another friend who was wearing -10 diopters. He wore his friend's glasses for a week before appearing before the military board. As one would expect, his vision was deemed below the necessary military standard and he was rejected.

He returned the glasses to his friend and his own eyes returned to normal. This story shows us just how much the eyesight can change over a small span of time. As mentioned earlier, there is no doubt that eyesight is influenced by external factors. Therefore, wearing lenses that are under-corrected by up to 1 diopter allows your eyes to adapt and change naturally during the course of the day.

Wearing under-corrected glasses does not in itself do much to improve your eyesight. It may slow the rate of deterioration but is unlikely to produce any dramatic improvement. However, under-corrected lenses, combined with Vision Training exercises, can actually become a Vision Training tool.

In the Renaissance, your eye-care specialist would lend you a pair of frames and keep reducing your lens prescription every three or four days until your vision was back to normal. I guess that one of those guys had an MBA from somewhere and discovered that you could actually keep people coming back every year for new glasses!

Apart from wearing under-prescribed lenses, there are two kinds of exercises that you need to do to help your eyes return to normal. Firstly, you need to do exercises that help get the energy back into your eyes, and secondly to do active exercises that train your eyes to extend their point of clarity outwards.

Under-correction

There are very few studies that examine the effect of under-correction. Tokoro and Kabe (1985, 1986) compared myopia progression rates during a three-year period for 33 children who entered school with low myopia. Thirteen of the children were given full correction and were instructed to wear glasses all the time. Ten children were under-corrected by 1 diopter or more. A further ten children were given full correction but told only to wear the glasses when necessary.

Gross (1994) calculated the myopia progress rates for the children not receiving pharmacological treatment and these 11 children were fully corrected on a full-time basis, the mean annual rate of myopia progression (±1 SD) was 0.83 diopters. However, for the five children who were under-corrected the mean annual rate of progression was only 0.47 diopters (±0.009 SD). So the myopia progression rate was cut almost in half.

From the above we can see that to simply under-correct is an effective means of arresting the progression of myopia. Simple under-correction is not sufficient to actually reverse the myopia, but combined with Vision Training myopia can be reversed. Of course this is easiest when there are only a few diopters of myopia.

Energy exercise

The eyes function as a part of the brain, consuming as much as 30 percent of the energy used by the brain when they observe an object. Therefore it is easy to understand that the eyes need an abundance of available free flowing energy. One of the consequences of myopia above just a few diopters is the lack of energy in the eyes. The Chinese call this life-giving energy chi.

This exercise is in two parts. First of all you remove the old, tired energy from your eyes and then you bring in a fresh source of vitality. The objective is to give your eyes plenty of energy so they can respond to Vision Training exercises with vigor. This exercise is the one that actually cured my eyesight, and is based on the pranic healing tradition developed by Master Choa Kok Sui.

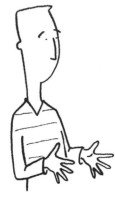

1. Activate your hands by gently touching the center of each palm with the opposite fingertip and then shake your hands vigorously.

2. Close the four fingers of your left or right hand, whichever you prefer, to form an imaginary arrow. Close your eyes and imagine soft apple-green energy flowing from the center of your palm down through your folded fingers in such a way that it creates a beam of this green energy.

    Raise your hand and direct this stream towards the energy center located between your eyebrows.

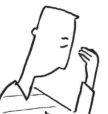

    Imagine that the energy flows in an endless stream from your fingertips into the point between your eyebrows and fills your eyes with cleansing apple-green energy. This should last for as long as it takes you to breathe in and out six to eight times. Then bring your hand down.

3. Next imagine that you are wearing a glove of transparent green or violet energy, which extends about 10 cm from your fingertips. Use your extended energy fingers to scoop away tired and old stress from your eyes. It is important that you clean the eyes all the way to the back of the eyeball. You will feel all the tiredness and tension being swept away from your eyes.

4. Now imagine lavender or pale violet energy flowing from your palm and direct this towards the energy point between your eyes. This lavender energy will re-energize your entire visual system. Once again do this as you count six or eight breathing cycles.

5. Turn your head to the left if you are right-handed. Find the energy point located at the back of your head at the same level as your eyes.

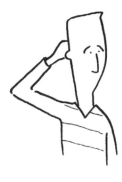

6. Project apple-green energy and briefly clean the energy center. Then project white energy into the back of your head and imagine this energy flowing from your fingertips into the back of your brain. This energizes the visual

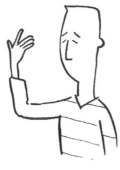

cortex located at the back of your head. Continue this process – energizing and flowing into the center of the brain – where it separates into two streams following and energizing the optic nerve and flowing into the back of the eyes – energizing the retina, the fovea, the muscles around the eyes, the lens, the cornea and the eyelids. Imagine your eyes filled with brilliant stimulating white light. Allow your intuition to guide you as to when you have had enough.

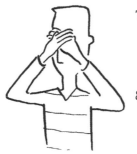

7. Imagine that your hand is a paint-roller dipped in sky-blue energy. With one or two sweeps, paint a layer of blue around the energy you have projected into your eyes. The blue will stabilize the energy.

8. Finally, rub your palms together until they get nice and warm. End the exercise with about 30 seconds of palming. You may see beautiful colors swirling around. This is the energy being absorbed into your system.

In the beginning I couldn't see the colors, so don't be concerned if you can't see them either. After a while this may start to change. In any case, remember that it is your intention that directs the energy and "energy follows thought." If you have difficulty imagining colors you could look at a sample of each color before visualizing it.

This exercise is very effective and will quickly restore vital energy to your eyes. Your eyes will feel clean and refreshed. The colors around you may seem brighter.

Note: It is possible to over-energize your eyes. You will feel as if your head has been stuffed! The remedy is to sweep the excess energy away, or go and lean against a tree. The tree will automatically balance your energy level.

For maximum benefit, do this exercise every two hours. Your first objective is to get enough energy into the eyes and for them to feel comfortable throughout the day. If you wear glasses with a power of more than 2 diopters you will have experienced how quickly your eyes tire whenever you remove them. Just like when a car battery goes flat, the car will start, but only after a couple of tries. The objective is first of all to restore an adequate level of energy to your eyes. Then you can develop additional energy so that your eyes are able to respond to the Vision Training exercises. Without energy in your eyes you won't get very far.

This exercise is the key to your myopia program. You should perform it every two hours until there is an adequate build-up of energy in your eyes. One of my participants in Manila, in the Philippines, was able to regain an impressive 3 diopters in only three days. She went from -6 diopters on Friday morning to -3 diopters on Sunday evening. To achieve this she practiced the exercise every half hour.

The energetic aspect of vision is not widely understood, and even less easy to comprehend is what can be done about it. In fact it is the key to regaining your eyesight. I have participants who have regained 5, 7 and even 8 diopters of myopia through this practice. The results have been objectively measured, with patients taking regular optometric tests to reduce their prescription.

String exercise

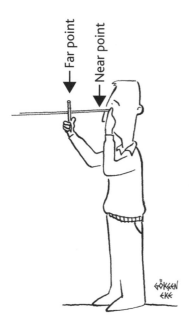

The string exercise is designed to give you a quantifiable method of measuring the parameters of your vision. Most people have difficulty understanding the meaning of a diopter reading. The string exercise provides definite and quantifiable feedback. All you need is a piece of string about 1.5 meters in length, a colored pen, a bookmark shaped piece of paper or card and a tape measure.

1. Firstly we need to measure the range of vision in each eye. This is done by placing one end of the string on the cheekbone, just below whichever eye you are testing. Tie the other end of the string to a chair or something convenient.

2. Use a bookmark shaped piece of paper or card that is inscribed with bright colors and large text. Slowly bring in the marker, holding it right next to the string, and starting from the other end of the string. Stop at the point where the text is no longer clearly visible.

It is important to emphasize the word clearly. We want the mind to understand that we want clear vision, so sending that message is of paramount importance.

Using one of the colored pens, mark this point on the string – the near point of absolutely clear vision. In most cases the near point is quite easy to identify. It should be less than 15 cm from your eyes.

3. Next, we want to find the point on the string where distance vision is no longer absolutely clear. You find that by slowly moving the marker out until the point where the text is no longer clear. Mark the far point of clear vision on the string. You now have a measure of the current extent of clear vision in that eye. The exercise thus far is just about providing a benchmark so that you can see how you progress. Now we come to the actual training part of the exercise.

4. Use one eye and follow the pen back and forth from about 5 cm before your far point where you can see it clearly and then out to about 5 cm beyond it, so your eyes begin to focus further and further away. Begin to involve your breathing. Exhale as you move your eyes outwards and inhale as you move your eyes back. Do this slowly. You will notice that your eyes start improving their ability to focus on the pen as it moves further and further away. You only need to do this exercise for 5 minutes at a time, but try to perform it ten times each day.

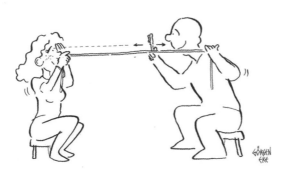

Distance to far point	Diopters
100 cm	-1.0
75 cm	-1.5
50 cm	-2.0
40 cm	-2.5
33 cm	-3.0
28 cm	-3.5
25 cm	-4.0
22.5 cm	-4.5
20 cm	-5.0
18 cm	-5.5
15 cm	-6.0
14 cm	-7.0
12.5 cm	-8.0
11 cm	-9.0
10 cm	-10.0

This string exercise is exceptionally effective for exercising your focusing ability – the medical term is *accommodation*. You have constant feedback as you progress. In fact, you can improve your vision quite dramatically doing this exercise. For example, if you have 5 diopters of eyesight, your far point will be about 20 cm from the end of the string. Follow the string back and forth from 5 cm before your far point to 5 cm beyond your far point. Once your ability to see the marker has improved enough to be able to see it 5 cm further away, you will have regained one full diopter of your eyesight.

Check both eyes and compare the near point and far points for each eye. The near point should be 15 cm or less from the end of the string. If you have a high degree of myopia, then the near point may be quite close to the end of the string. If this is the case, there is no need to be concerned about it. On the other hand if the near point is more than 15 cm away then you are developing presbyopia or "old eyes." This is usually not an issue if you are near-sighted.

Compare your far points. They should be exactly the same. If there is a difference, then you have anisometropic vision (i.e., one eye that has better vision than the other). This is the condition you need to attend to first. If left alone you could develop amblyopia in the weaker eye. This means that your brain simply switches off the input from that eye. Often people are not aware of this since it develops very slowly.

To correct the imbalance between your eyes use the string exercise and work with the weaker eye until both eyes are the same. The string exercise is a superb tool for restoring vision in an amblyopic eye.

Coming and going exercise

Assuming that myopia is a functional and learned phenomena, I have for years been looking for an exercise for myopia that would be equally effective as the Tibetan wheel exercise is for astigmatism. The main problem in myopia is that the oblique muscles hold too much tension, combined with what ophthalmologists would call *excessive accommodation* (i.e., the ciliary muscle around the lens is in a constant state of tension). This is the all too common experience of trying to see things in the distance clearly, especially after you have been using a computer. In other words, you are straining to see.

When you have a stiff shoulder or neck you begin to move your shoulder and head so the muscle is stretched and thereby releases the tension. This is one of the fundamental principles of all bodywork approaches. The question is: How do you exercise and relax the two oblique muscles in the eye?

The eye muscles work in pairs and are all involved in any movement. However, the active force of turning the eyes is performed by pairs of muscles. It is a fluid relationship that exists between pulling and holding. This dynamic enables the fluid movement of your eyes as you track the flight of a bird from one tree to another or in reading this page. Normally, this process happens quite naturally and without any effort. However, if for one reason or another you happen to hold too much tension in one or more of your eye muscles, they will automatically exert undue pressure on the eyeball and cause undesirable stress patterns. The research done by Peter Greene (1980, 1981) using mechanical engineering principles in studying myopia, shows that tension held by the oblique muscles creates a higher level of stress on the back of the eyes where, in cases of myopia, an elongation is apparent.

Looking at the way that eye muscles work, I have noticed that the obliques are most engaged when you turn the eyes inwards towards the tip of your nose. The coming and going exercise is designed to stretch your oblique muscles and is especially beneficial for people with myopia.

The movements of this exercise are done at the center line right in front of you. Keep your head still and only move your eyes.

1. Take a pen or use one of your fingers and begin to slowly move it from below, and close to your body, up towards the tip of your nose. While looking at the pen, continue the movement until the pen actually touches the tip of your nose and your eyes are turned in towards your nose.

2. Next, very slowly begin to move the pen out horizontally in front of you. Keep looking at the pen as it moves out to arm's length. Now, look out in the distance beyond the pen. Look around and notice what you see. It does not matter if it's clear or not. What matters is that you send signals to your brain that you want to see further into the distance.

    Shift back to looking at the pen and begin to move it slowly back towards the tip of your nose. Continue to look at the pen until it physically touches the tip of your nose.

3. Next, begin to move the pen up while you follow with your eyes. This is the going movement. Finally, move the pen back down and touch the tip of your nose.

4. Continue doing these movements very slowly, keeping it fluid and easy. Do this a total of perhaps five times. Notice what happens to your eye muscles. If they get sore, then stop for a while and then take up the exercise again. The

coming and going exercise is good for any kind of myopia and can be combined with other exercises as appropriate.

After doing this exercise you will most probably feel that the muscles at the back of your eyes have been given a workout. Be careful not to over-exert the oblique muscles. If you feel sore then stop doing the exercise. You can do this exercise in most places without drawing too much attention to yourself. The higher the degree of myopia you have, the more important this exercise is.

17. Presbyopia

Presbyopia, the need for reading glasses, afflicts a lot of people when they reach their mid-forties. The first sign you notice may be that you start to have difficulty reading in low light – for example, reading menus in dimly lit restaurants. Then you might find that you are experiencing difficulty in reading small print. You may need to hold the text further and further away until your arms are just not long enough to hold the book in the right position. You could also find yourself squinting, but unfortunately it doesn't help very much.

Regrettably optometrists will often decide that you need reading glasses when you reach your forties. I know of many cases where patients were not even tested but just told that they should consider getting bifocal glasses. The automatic assumption that you lose your ability to read without glasses when you reach your mid-forties is an unfortunate mass belief that all too many people buy into.

The decline in eyesight is so linear that tables have been made correlating vision with a person's age. At age 10 you have about 20 diopters of focusing ability. You are expected to have lost half of your original accommodative power by age 30, and by the age of 40 to be missing about two thirds. Less than 5 diopters of accommodation or focusing ability is considered to be presbyopia. At age 60 your focusing powers are presumed to be practically non-existent. Eye-care professionals consider presbyopia to be present in virtually 100 percent of people over 50. Fortunately this does not actually reflect reality.

There are two main theories that endeavor to explain presbyopia. The influential German scientist Helmholtz (1866) suggested that presbyopia was caused by a hardening of the lens, and Dutch ophthalmologist Donders (1864) attributed presbyopia to a weakening of the ciliary muscle fibers in which the lens is suspended. During the last 135 years there has been very little progress in this field, since these are the same explanations most eye-care professionals will offer today.

However, not everyone agrees. Researchers Saladin et al. (1974) published a paper in which they investigated the strength of the ciliary muscle. They discovered that this muscle actually continued to contract after accommodation was achieved, suggesting that it had additional strength and could be contracted even further. Tamm et al. (1992) postulated that the ciliary muscle force should not reach zero until the age of 120.

My experience with presbyopia leads me to believe that it is very easy to correct. One of the many success stories I have about eliminating the need for reading glasses is that of a good friend of mine whom I visited in Illinois one summer. She had been diagnosed as needing reading glasses a few months before, but as I was coming to give a Vision Training course she did not actually go out and buy them. In fact, I did not know at the time that she needed glasses. As I was working with some of her friends, she picked up what to do and to this day reads perfectly without glasses. The thing to do is to move your eyes from small details, like very small print, to large print and look at things in the medium distance as well as looking far away. This habit keeps the eyes flexible and means that you can expect to be able to read comfortably for a long time.

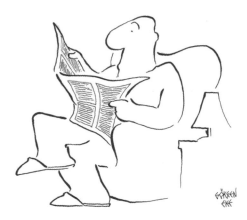

Another example of how easily presbyopia can be corrected involves a friend of a professor of ophthalmology who was wearing reading glasses. As a joke, I invited him to join the professor when he visited my vision class the following day – on the condition that he learn how to read without his glasses. The next day at the workshop I introduced him to reading progressively smaller and smaller print. To the astonishment of the professor, his friend was able to read tiny print in about 10 minutes. Reading tiny print is far beyond what you would normally expect to be required to read. The following year the professor shared with a group of ophthalmologists that the presbyopia exercise he learned that day had resulted in a reduction of 50 percent in his sale of reading glasses. Interestingly enough, his patient ratio had also gone up during the year he had shared the Vision Training exercises with his patients.

During an evening workshop in Cork, Ireland I met a boy of 14 who had been wearing plus lenses for eight years (more than half his life). I told him that the world record for learning to read without glasses was 15 minutes. If he wanted to he could break that record and I would mention him in my workshops all over the world. He accomplished this feat in 10 minutes, working with the exercise of reading progressively smaller and smaller print.

The way I think about presbyopia is that as we grow older our muscles become less flexible. We are not as agile at 45 as we were at 15 or 25. This of course also applies to the eye muscles. So what is called for, it seems, are some tai chi type exercises for the eyes. The technique of reading progressively smaller and smaller print is extremely effective.

William H. Bates, the grandfather of Vision Training, writes an interesting story about how he discovered the cure for presbyopia in an article in *Better Eyesight* in 1922.

Bates' road to discovering the cure for presbyopia

Dr. Bates writes about an incident that happened in around 1912 when a friend asked him to read a letter. To his embarrassment, Bates had to spend some time searching for his reading glasses.

> Being a friend he could say things no other person would say. Among the disagreeable things he said was, and the tone was very empathetic, sarcastic, disagreeable, insulting, "You claim to cure people without glasses; why don't you cure yourself?" I shall never forget those words. They stimulated me to do something. I tried all manner of means, by concentration, strain, effort, hard work, to enable myself to become able to read the newspaper at the near point ... I consulted specialists in hypnotism, electricity experts, neurologists of all kinds and many others. One I called on, a physician who was an authority in psychoanalysis, was kind enough to listen to my problem. With as few words as possible I explained to him the simple method by which we diagnose nearsightedness with the retinoscope.
>
> As I looked off into the distance, he examined my eyes, and said that they were normal, but when I made an effort to see at a distance he said that my eyes were focused for the reading distance, i.e. nearsighted. Then when I looked at fine print

at the reading distance and tried to read it, he said that my eyes were focused for a distance of twenty feet or farther, and the harder I tried to read, the farther away I pushed my focus. He was convinced of the facts, namely: a strain to see at the distance produced nearsightedness, while a strain to see near produced a farsighted eye ...

Stumbling on the truth

The man who finally helped me to succeed, or rather the only man who would do anything to encourage me, was an Episcopal minister living in Brooklyn. After my evening office hours I had to travel for about two hours to reach his residence. With the aid of the retinoscope, while I was making all kinds of efforts to focus my eyes at the near point, he would tell me how well I was succeeding. After some weeks or months I had made no progress.

But one night I was looking at a picture on the wall, which had black spots in different parts of it. They were conspicuously black. While observing them my mind imagined they were dark caves and that there were people moving around in them. My friend told me my eyes were now focused at the near point. When I tried to read my eyes were now focused for the distance.

Lying on the table in front of me was a magazine with an illustrated advertisement with black spots which were intensely black. I imagined they were openings of caves with people moving around in them. My friend told me that my eyes were focused for the near point; and when I glanced at some reading matter, I was able to read it. Then I looked at a newspaper and while doing so remembered the perfect black of my imaginary caves and was gratified to find that I was able to read perfectly.

We discussed the matter to find what brought about the benefit. Was it strain, or what was it? I tried again to

The drifting near point

As you grow older the eye muscles become less flexible and the near point of clear vision tends to drift out. Below is an approximate scale of the average near point of clear vision vs. age.

Age	Distance
50	40 cm
Normal reading distance	35 cm
40	20 cm
30	14 cm
20	10 cm
10	7 cm

remember the black caves while looking at the newspaper and my memory failed. I could not read the newspaper at all. He asked, "Do you remember the black caves?" I answered, "No, I don't seem to be able to remember the black caves. "Well," he said, "close your eyes and remember the black caves." And when I opened my eyes I was able to read – for a few moments. When I tried to remember the black caves again I failed.

The harder I tried, the less I succeeded and we were puzzled. We discussed the matter and talked of a number of things, and all of a sudden without an effort on my part I remembered the black caves, and sure enough, it helped me to read. We talked some more. Why did I fail to remember the black caves when I tried so hard? Why did I remember the black caves when I did not try or while I was thinking of other things? Here was a problem. We were both very interested and finally it dawned on me that I could only remember these black caves when I did not strain or make an effort.

I had discovered the truth: *a perfect memory is obtained without effort and in no other way*. Also, *when the memory or imagination is perfect, sight is perfect*. (Bates, 1922; emphasis in original)

Presbyopia is due to stress not age. Consequently, if the stress and strain are relieved, the ability to read and see at the near point comes back.

Vision Training principles for presbyopia

- Bring the near point of clear focus in to about 15 cm from the eyes.

- Develop relaxation in the eye muscles so they can stretch and contract to their full ability. This is done with a simple exercise involving reading progressively smaller and smaller print.

- Train your eyes to function in a variety of light sources.

- Encourage your eyes' ability to converge on the paper of the book or magazine you are reading.

From a Vision Training point of view, we think of presbyopia as a result of an overall loss of flexibility in muscle tone. When you were 18 you could go out dancing all night and still go to work or school the next day without too much trouble. By the age of 45 you have lost some of that flexibility and your muscles are just not that supple. The same thing is happening with your eyes. In order to regain your reading ability, therefore, you need to stretch and soften your eye muscles so they can regain the range of accommodation you need for good reading.

In order to restore comfortable reading ability you need to do some simple exercises. These are designed to get your eyes to relax and allow the eye muscles to gradually stretch and thereby increase your ability to read. Generally you will want to practice until you can comfortably read really small print. This way you will have spare capacity so you will be able to read labels in the supermarket, even when you are tired, or read the phone book in moonlight, should you ever need that ability.

Nowadays we have access to adequate lighting 24 hours a day, so we tend not to use our low light vision as much as we would if there was no electric lighting at night. Your eyes use a different set of light sensitive cells for detecting low light (rod cells) than for bright light and color images (cone cells). So, to train your ability to read under different light sources, I recommend that you experiment with all sorts of light levels until you can read really small print with just one candle. In this way you will regain your ability to see well in any light conditions.

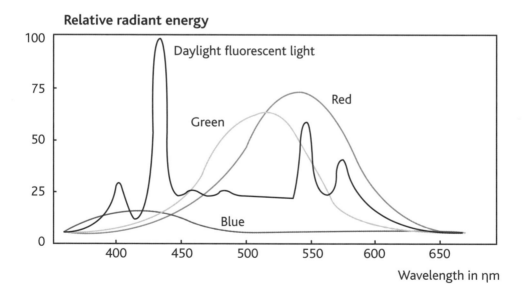

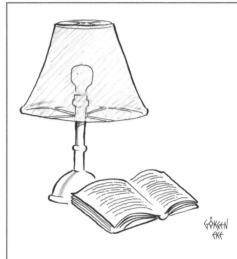

Good reading light

A study was carried out comparing the visual effects of different lights on the printed page. Sunshine reflected from a white printed page at noon on a clear day registers at 1,300 foot candles (1 foot candle is the light from one candle at the distance of 1 foot). In an outdoor shadow the reflection is reduced to 130 foot candles.

Indoors, a 150-watt reflector spot bulb registers at 130 foot candles, the same reading as in shadow outdoors on a sunny day. A 60-watt bulb at the same distance registers only 2 foot candles, reflected from the same page. Indirect light by a 300-watt bulb thrown off the ceiling measures only half a foot candle. Fluorescent light registered about a quarter of a foot candle.

No wonder fluorescent light is so tiring.

The worst light source you can use for work or reading is fluorescent light tubes, which typically produce a rather distorted spectrum of light. For example, cool-white fluorescent light, the most frequently used, is deficient in red and blue-violet colors, the area where natural sunlight is strongest. Also, fluorescent light casts very few shadows. These are important for the eye in order to determine shape. In uniform light your brain has to work harder to detect the shape of objects. In addition, fluorescent tubes contain only half of the colors compared to daylight and they also tend to flicker, thus leading to eyestrain. This is especially prevalent in areas where the level of power supply fluctuates.

If you are working in an environment where there is nothing but fluorescent light, I suggest that you add a table lamp with an incandescent or halogen light. This will blend with the colors emitted from the fluorescent tubes and produce a better environment for your eyes. You will feel the difference very quickly. Often I have to conduct seminars in rooms where there is only fluorescent light. People begin to develop eyestrain after just a few hours in this environment. Consequently, I always specify seminar rooms with good daylight. There is nothing better, and it's free.

Another problem is convergence (the ability to focus both eyes on the same point). Often one eye will be focusing on the paper while the other actually focuses a few centimeters in front and behind the page causing you to get tired easily. In some cases people have what is known as mono-vision, where you use one eye for reading and one eye for seeing at a distance. To correct for convergence at the reading distance we use convergence charts that train your eyes to fuse the images from both eyes into one three-dimensional image.

Do you have presbyopia?

If you have 20/20 vision for reading then you should be able to read these lines in good daylight using the normal reading distance:

20/50	A b C d E f G h I j K 1 3 5 7 9 2 4 6 8
20/40	A b C d E f G h I j K 1 3 5 7 9 2 4 6 8
20/30	A b C d E f G h I j K 1 3 5 7 9 2 4 6 8 Your reading vision may be OK for most situations; however, you may have difficulty in low light situations.
20/25	A b C d E f G h I j K 1 3 5 7 9 2 4 6 8 Your reading vision is pretty good. Just a fraction below the optimum.
20/20	Judgment is the summation, the end result, the interpretation or evaluation of what the eye sees.
20/16	A b C d E f G h I j K 1 3 5 7 9 2 4 6 8 Congratulations you have perfect near-point reading vision.

The numbers in the left column are the Snellen indicators. Note that the quality of light has a great influence on your reading ability. Indoors in the evening your visual acuity for reading will drift up a line or two. Ideally you should be able to see the 20/20 line, crystal clearly, at about 15–20 cm in front of your eyes. This is normal visual acuity for activities at the near point. Children can see this print at about 10 cm in front of their eyes.

Small print exercise

Dr. William Bates maintained that it was impossible to read fine print without relaxing the visual system. Therefore the reading of such print, contrary to what is generally believed, is of great benefit to the eyes.

Simply bring the fine print so near to the eyes that it cannot be read. Of course you realize that you can't read this close and your eyes do not even try to see, and then relax. Alternately open and close your eyes for a few seconds while looking at the fine print and notice what happens.

People whose sight is beginning to fail at the near point or who are approaching the so-called presbyopic age, should imitate the example of a remarkable old gentleman I met. Get a sample of really small print and read it a few times every day. Start in good daylight then in different kinds of artificial light, bringing it closer and closer to the eye until it can be read at about 15 centimetres or less. Or get a sample of type reduced by photography until it is much smaller, and do the same. You will thus escape, not only the necessity of wearing glasses for reading and near work, but all those eye troubles which now so often afflict people. Nature intended that you should have natural clear eyesight.

This exercise should be done with good daylight illuminating the page. Before reading the text below, remove your reading glasses and rest your eyes for a few minutes by palming. Then turn the page upside down and proceed to scan the white space between the lines and as you do so imagine that the background is brilliantly white like sunlight reflected on water or snow. Keep your breathing nice and deep. Continue to scan the white spaces as if you were reading. Go all the way to the bottom of the page. Now turn the book right side up and notice how many more words or paragraphs you can read.

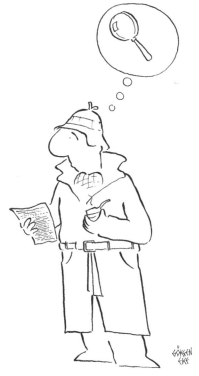

There is no need to read each paragraph – it's the same text in different font sizes. Continue this exercise for 5 minutes or until you can read to the bottom paragraph. That is, read it from any distance within arm's length. You will first notice that words appear to become clear, then sentences and finally the whole paragraph will be clear. For some people this process is very rapid but for others they need to practice a few times before they relax enough to allow their eyes to adjust. It is about allowing yourself to explore the possibility of developing more flexibility and discovering how it would look and feel. It is an intriguing question, isn't it? How would I feel if I could read print this small?

Persons whose sight is beginning to fail at the near point, or who are approaching the so-called presbyopic age, should imitate the example of a remarkable old gentleman I met. Find a sample of really small print and

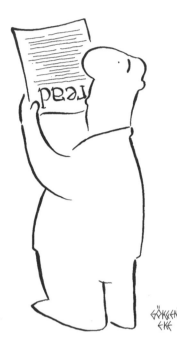

read it a few times every day. Start in good daylight then in different kinds of artificial light, bringing it closer and closer to the eye until it can be read at about 15 cm or less. Or get a sample of type reduced until it is much smaller, and do the same. You will thus escape not only the necessity of wearing glasses for reading, but all those eye troubles which so often afflict people. Nature intended that you should have natural clear eyesight.

Persons whose sight is beginning to fail at the near point or who are approaching the so-called presbyopic age, should imitate the example of a remarkable old gentleman I met. Find a sample of really small print and read it a few times every day. Start in good daylight then in different kinds of artificial light, bringing it closer and closer to the eye until it can be read at about 15 cm or less. Or get a sample of type reduced until it is much smaller, and do the same. You will thus escape not only the necessity of wearing glasses for reading, but all those eye troubles which so often afflict people. Nature intended that you should have natural clear eyesight.

Persons whose sight is beginning to fail at the near point or who are approaching the so-called presbyopic age, should imitate the example of a remarkable old gentleman I met. Find a sample of really small print and read it a few times every day. Start in good daylight then in different kinds of artificial light, bringing it closer and closer to the eye until it can be read at about 15 cm or less. Or get a sample of type reduced until it is much smaller, and do the same. You will thus escape not only the necessity of wearing glasses for reading, but all those eye troubles which so often afflict people. Nature intended that you should have natural clear eyesight.

Persons whose sight is beginning to fail at the near point or who are approaching the so-called presbyopic age, should imitate the example of a remarkable old gentleman. Find a sample of really small print and read it a few times every day. Start in good daylight then in different kinds of artificial light, bringing it closer and closer to the eye until it can be read at about 15 cm or less. Or get a sample of type reduced until it is much smaller, and do the same. You will thus escape not only the necessity of wearing glasses for reading, but all those eye troubles which so often afflict people. Nature intended that you should have natural clear eyesight.

Persons whose sight is beginning to fail at the near point or who are approaching the so-called presbyopic age, should imitate the example of a remarkable old gentleman. Find a sample of really small print and read it a few times every day. Start in good daylight then in different kinds of artificial light, bringing it closer and closer to the eye until it can be read at about 15 cm or less. Or get a sample of type reduced until it is much smaller, and do the same. You will thus escape not only the necessity of wearing glasses for reading, but all those eye troubles which so often afflict people. Nature intended that you should have natural clear eyesight.

Persons whose sight is beginning to fail at the near point or who are approaching the so-called presbyopic age, should imitate the example of a remarkable old gentleman I met. Find a sample of really small print and read it a few times every day. Start in good daylight then in different kinds of artificial light, bringing it closer and closer to the eye until it can be read at about 15 cm or less. Or get a sample of type reduced by photography until it is much smaller, and do the same. You will thus escape not only the necessity of wearing glasses for reading, but all those eye troubles which so often afflict people. Nature intended that you should have natural clear eyesight.

Persons whose sight is beginning to fail at the near point or who are approaching the so-called presbyopic age, should imitate the example of a remarkable old gentleman I met. Find a sample of really small print and read it a few times every day. Start in good daylight then in different kinds of artificial light, bringing it closer and closer to the eye until it can be read at about 15 cm or less. Or get a sample of type reduced by photography until it is much smaller, and do the same. You will thus escape not only the necessity of wearing glasses for reading, but all those eye troubles which so often afflict people. Nature intended that you should have natural clear eyesight.

Persons whose sight is beginning to fail at the near point or who are approaching the so-called presbyopic age, should imitate the example of a remarkable old gentleman I met. Find a sample of really small print and read it a few times every day. Start in good daylight then in different kinds of artificial light, bringing it closer and closer to the eye until it can be read at about 15 cm or less. Or get a sample of type reduced by photography until it is much smaller, and do the same. You will thus escape not only the necessity of wearing glasses for reading and near work, but all those eye troubles which now so often afflict people. Nature intended that you should have natural clear eyesight.

Persons whose sight is beginning to fail at the near point or who are approaching the so-called presbyopic age, should imitate the example of a remarkable old gentleman I met. Find a sample of really small print and read it a few times every day. Start in good daylight then in different kinds of artificial light, bringing it closer and closer to the eye until it can be read at about 15 cm or less. Or get a sample of type reduced by photography until it is much smaller, and do the same. You will thus escape not only the necessity of wearing glasses for reading and near work, but all those eye troubles which now so often afflict people. Nature intended that you should have natural clear eyesight.

Congratulations, if you can read this comfortably with both artificial light and in daylight then you have 20/20 near vision. To maintain your near vision you need to read small print like this or smaller at least a few times every month. Take something you are really interested in reading and use a photocopying machine and have the magazine or article reduced to small print like this. Then read it with regular light and with just one candle. You can have a glass of wine as a reward. When you are reading with the absolute minimum light possible, you are training your visual system to function comfortably with very low light. Now go and find the darkest spot in the room and read this again. How did it go? Now do this about once a week from now on and your eyesight will be fine for the rest of your life.

If you can read this in daylight then you have perfect near vision. Most people can only read this small print with sunlight. Keep playing with your ability to read really small print and you will also maintain your optimum near-point visual acuity.

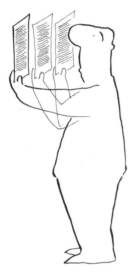

The next step is to check if there is a difference between your two eyes. Look at one of the small print paragraphs that you can comfortably read. Close your left eye. If you need to move the book there is a difference between your eyes. Now, switch the eyes and look at the small print with your right eye. Again, if you need to move the book there is a difference.

To equalize the reading distance between your two eyes, close the near eye. Move the book to the point where the eye that read the furthest away can see the text clearly. To encourage the eye to adjust, begin to move the book just a little bit closer so the text starts to become blurred. The eye will now attempt to adjust for the slight difference and in most cases succeed in doing so. Continue this backwards and forwards movement until your eyes can read at the same level.

Finally, you will want to train your eyes to read in a variety of light conditions. In bright daylight the cone cells are active and provide you with crystal clear vision. In low light you will need to use more of the rod cells which are highly sensitive to light. You naturally move from one type of cell to another and have the ability to read small print in very low light conditions. This is similar to reading the phone book in moonlight as mentioned above. Train your eyes to be able to easily read multicolored menus in dimly lit restaurants.

When you can read the above paragraph in good daylight then progress to read it in lower and lower light. Step inside the room and notice how this changes your ability to read. Continue to find different light levels until you can read fine print with just one candle.

Lazy reading exercise

The purpose of this exercise is to develop flexibility in focusing between the near point and far point and sharpening your focusing powers. This exercise also develops the ability to read smoothly without regressing

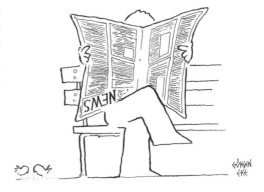

1. Find a book or a magazine printed with plenty of white space between the lines and a typeface that appears slightly blurred when you hold the page up in front of you.

2. Turn the page upside down so that you cannot read the text.

3. Run your eyes gently and slowly around the margins a few times, looking as if from the back of your head.

4. Now choose two points at the top corners of the page, and another, such as a box of tissues, at a distance within the room.

5. Shift your eyes from the page to the box and back and forth.

6. Next, scan the white spaces between the lines, going down the page as if you were reading. By the time you are halfway down, everything may seem clearer, but do not strive for clarity, keep going.

7. When you reach the bottom, turn the book or magazine right side up, and look along the white space below the first line of type.

8. Close your eyes now, and from memory paint imaginary white in the space below the first line of type, back and forth.

9. Open your eyes and scan the spaces beneath the first few lines, imagining them as being bright as snow in brilliant sunlight. Repeat this several times, alternately closing and opening your eyes.

10. Now float your eyes back and forth over the lines without reading.

11. Look away then return to the page. The black of the type will seem blacker and the white of the spaces will seem whiter than you have ever seen them. The words will stand out sharply.

Devote 15 minutes a day to this exercise. In the weeks to follow gradually reduce the size of type with which you are practicing until you are able to easily <small>read small print</small> .

Circle exercise

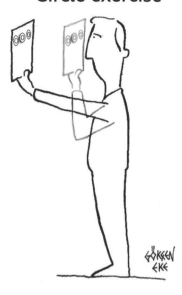

This exercise will teach your centering muscles to work in partnership with your focusing muscles. Usually when your eye-crossing muscle lacks tone, you will automatically over-focus and your near point is pushed out beyond the page you are reading. This can lead to presbyopia and astigmatism.

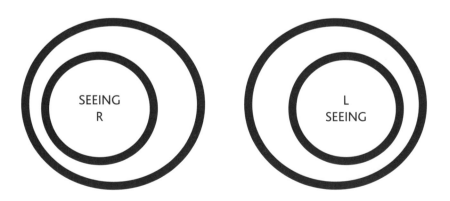

Position this page so the circles are very close to your eyes. The left and right circles will float together and form a three-dimensional image in the center. The inner circle now floats above the outer circle like a multilayered cake. The word SEEING floats on top and you will see two words one above the other.

If you see the "R" and the "L" that means your fusion is not quite complete. The perfect alignment shows the word SEEING in two lines, perfectly aligned one above the other. No "R" and no "L" are seen. Keep this image and slowly move the book away from you until it is at arm's length. You should be able to maintain the fusion and the image in perfect focus at all distances from about 15 cm to arm's length. Next look away and back again. You should be able to get the fused image back instantly. Practice for a few minutes at a time and frequently until you get the image. If you notice that your eye muscles are becoming sore then stop the exercise. This is about developing flexibility, so be gentle.

Hold the diagram at your normal reading distance and begin to slowly move the page in clockwise circles, progressively making larger and larger circles. Do the same in a counter-clockwise direction. This will train your ability to keep fusion all over the printed page.

Eventually you should be able to get the perfect fusion from close, up to arm's length, as well as being able to look away at something in the distance then switch back and get the perfectly fused image instantaneously. Once you can do that you can stop doing the circle exercises.

This is what you should see.

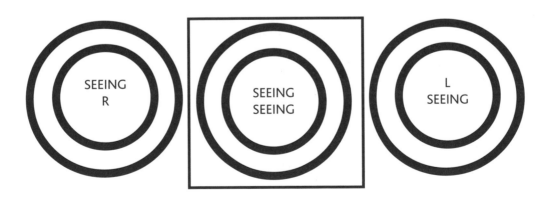

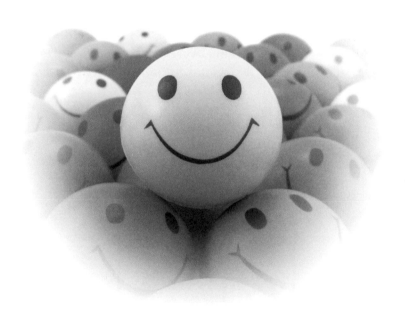

18. Hyperopia

Hyperopia or far-sight is common in young children. As the name suggests, your vision is good but near activities cause discomfort. Research indicates that most infants are about 1 diopter hyperopic. However, the natural process of growing up normalizes the vision and only about 10 percent of children still have hyperopia during their school years.

Hyperopia has been associated with reading and learning problems. For example, in 1989 Rosner and Rosner compared the visual characteristics of children who had difficulties in school. Surprisingly they found that 54 percent of them were hyperopic. Looking at the children who did well in school, they found more than half of them were myopic and 16 percent were hyperopic. Rosner looked at 710 schoolchildren aged from 6 to 12 years. He found significant visual analysis difficulties in as many as 82 percent of the children with hyperopia, whilst only 14 percent of the children with myopia had visual analysis problems.

The reading problems associated with hyperopia are generally attributed to the extra demand that leads to mental strain while reading. Consequently, children tend to avoid this activity as much as possible. In addition the near-point convergence becomes stressed.

It is easy to imagine how vision problems and learning go hand in hand. Having difficulty in learning links systemically with many other aspects of the life of a child. Tension held in the eyes, which is the root cause of hyperopia, is perhaps a response to holding off or maintaining stability in a situation where things may be very confusing.

Eye-care professionals have two main approaches to hyperopia in children. One school of thought prescribes plus lenses in order to relieve the eyestrain. They feel that hyperopia, if left untreated, may lead to binocular difficulties like amblyopia or strabismus (Ingram et al., 1986). The other school of thought discourages the use of lenses even with refraction errors as high as +7 diopters (Raab, 1982). The rationale is that children's ability to focus their eyes is far in excess of what is required to cope with hyperopia.

This of course poses a dilemma for parents as one doctor will say, "Don't use glasses" whilst another will say, "If you don't use glasses then this and that will happen." It is best that plus lenses should not be prescribed until a child demonstrates a "need" for them. These children have no difficulty in reading the blackboard, but when reading close-up they develop eyestrain, headaches, inability to focus for a long time and even behavioural problems.

Hyperopia (far-sightedness) is different from presbyopia which develops as you grow older, typically around the mid-forties.

From a Vision Training point of view, we use exercises that develop the near-focus ability of the eye. This is mainly a muscle exercise which produces excellent results.

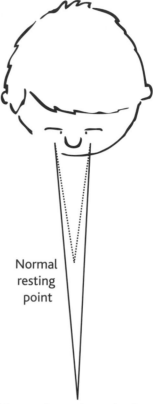

Normal resting point

Hyperopic resting point is further away

Vision Training principles for hyperopia

- Encourage relaxation of the entire visual system.

- Make sure the near point of clear vision is no more than 15 cm from the eyes.

- Read small print regularly.

There are several ways you can relax your eyes. The simple Bates exercise of palming is an excellent way to do this. Simply rub your hands together as you would on a cold winter day. When your palms are nice and warm, place your hands over your closed eyes. Your hands should be held so your palms are directly over the eyes. Your fingers do not have much effect. The warmth from your hands as well as the polarity difference between your hands and eyes results in you relaxing your eyes.

Another excellent way to relax your eyes, and possibly to reduce wrinkle lines around them, is to place teabags on your closed eyelids. The temperature should be so that it is pleasantly warm. Chamomile tea is an excellent choice because the chamomile has soothing properties as well.

Alternating hot and cold towels over the closed eyes is another effective way to relax them. When you fly long distance flights attendants will offer you hot towels when it is time for you to wake up. Placing the hot towel over your closed eyes washes away the tiredness from them. The cold towel will activate your blood circulation in the same way a cold shower does after a hot sauna. Do this a couple of times and you will experience a new vitality in your eyes.

Remember, in the case of hyperopia you already have the ability to focus close-up, so you just need to exercise that ability. Take every opportunity you can during the day to examine the smallest detail you can see at as close a range as possible. When I work with children I tell them to go and look in the eyes of ants, at the minute structure of a wall, the bark of a tree and so on. The goal is to exercise your ability to focus at the near point so it no longer requires so much effort. You will find that after a few days of doing this you can read for much longer periods without discomfort.

Dr. William Bates maintained that if you practice reading small print regularly then you will also maintain your natural clear eyesight. When you are able to read really small print then you are using your central foveal vision perfectly and it is impossible to strain your eyes doing that.

Here is the same paragraph this time printed in 3-point letters.

Dr. William Bates maintained that if you practice reading small print regularly then you will also maintain your natural clear eyesight. When you are able to read really small print then you are using your central foveal vision perfectly and it is impossible to strain your eyes doing that.

Read it in good daylight. What does it feel like to read this small print? How close-up can you read it clearly?

Practice reading as close as possible to your eyes. The normal near point of clear vision should be about 15 cm from your eyes. Move your reading material back and forth so your eyes begin to refocus at a closer and closer distance. With this simple trombone movement you are actually exercising your ability to read close-up.

You will notice an improvement almost right away. Keep doing the exercises until it becomes very easy for you to focus close-up and read comfortably for extended periods of time. After that, practice some of the exercises once in a while to keep your near focusing ability in top form.

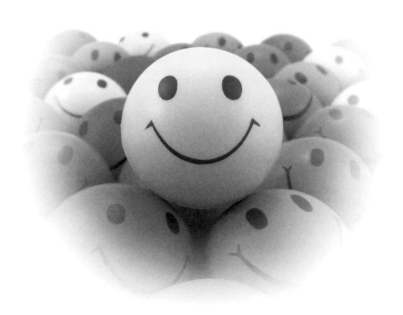

19. Convergence

The eyes of people with good vision naturally point to and converge at the object of interest. That is, the eyes rotate slightly so that the central fovea, where vision is clearest, is pointed directly at what you are looking at. The medical term for this is vergence function. You have probably noticed how the eyes turn inward when someone is looking at something very close-up, for instance when threading a needle. The eyes automatically turn in to keep the needle and thread in sharp focus. On the other hand, when someone is looking at a landscape the eyes seem to point almost straight ahead. Your eyes have this marvelous ability to always keep anything you want to see in sharp focus. Your eyes can watch a skier rushing down a mountainside and still keep the figure in focus while the background rushes by.

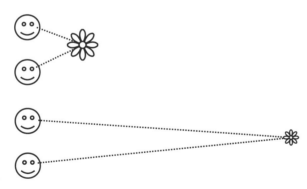

With proper convergence you have depth perception and experience the world in 3D. The brain automatically fuses the image from your left and right eye together into three-dimensional perception. You instantly know where things are located. Good depth perception is very important if you play ballgames where you need to catch a ball. If your convergence is off, you tend to misjudge where the ball will fall. Either you attempt to catch it short or the ball will fly over your head. Lack of convergence, or stereovision, usually does not affect reading. People with mono-vision using only one eye generally develop alternate ways of approximating distance, for example, by judging the size of objects.

It is believed that stereoscopic vision is developed by the age of 4 months and will be fully established around 8 years of age. Generally it is assumed that the entire visual system is fully developed by this age.

Severe convergence problems develop when one of the eyes turns in, as in esotropia or when one of the eyes turn out, as is the case in exotropia. This condition is known as strabismus. When the image from one eye crosses the midline of the retina, this operates as a trigger and the brain suspends the image from that eye in order to avoid double vision or diplopia.

To illustrate this phenomenon, look at something at a distance. Now, put your index finger in between yourself and the object. How many fingers do you see? Look at your finger – what happens to the object you were looking at? When you look at something in the distance anything in between will seem to double because the eyes are converged towards (pointing to) a more distant object. The foreground will be slightly out of focus.

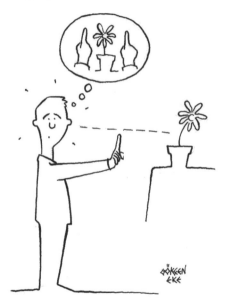

Natural convergence can slowly drift out of alignment. This happens very slowly and you probably will not notice this until you get your eyes tested. Convergence issues often play a role in vision problems. If your eyes are always converging slightly in front of what you actually want to see, then your eyes are over-converged and your vision will be out of focus – especially in low light. In environments where your pupils are opened widely, your depth of field will be very shallow. In bright light your pupils will be very small and your depth of field will be very large, resulting in a sharper image. The world will appear much clearer on a bright summer day.

Vision Training principles for convergence

- Practice the string exercise on page 124 which is designed to provide feedback as to when you have convergence.

- Practice moving the convergence to the point of attention. This is to correct for convergence ahead or behind the object you are looking at.

- Check that you have convergence at both near and far viewing distance.

From a Vision Training point of view convergence is quite easy to correct using a piece of string as a feedback device. We use an optical illusion that takes place when you are looking down a string with both of your eyes open. If you have perfect convergence you will see a phantom cross with its center right at the object you are looking at. The center of the cross will be where you focused your attention on the string.

How to test for convergence

Fusion is one of the easiest things to check and correct. Take a piece of string, about the length from hand to hand stretched across your chest (about 1.25 meters). Tie the string to the back of a chair or to a door handle. Next you will need a paperclip or a bead, which you can move up and down the string.

1. Place the loose end of the string on the tip of your nose so the string is stretched out.

2. Place the paperclip on the string somewhere in the middle.

3. When you look at the paperclip you should see two phantom lines crossing directly through the paperclip. If you see the cross in front of the paperclip then your eyes are under-converging. If you see the cross beyond the paperclip then your eyes are over-converging. If you see only one string, then one eye is suppressing the image. The brain is only attending to one image and is blocking the affected eye – you are only using one eye. Any misalignment contributes to your vision problem and makes images blurry.

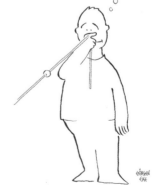

In some cases the outer eye muscles are too tight and refuse to allow the eyes to move in. If this is the case, then practice looking at your finger while you move it in from arm's length to physically touching the tip of your nose. When looking at something up-close, your eyes move in towards the nose.

Aligning your fusion point is easy. Simply move the paperclip in or out until it coincides with the cross point of the "X." In some cases people see a "V," others perceive it as more like an "A" and some people see the phenomenon more like a "Y." Any of these are fine as long as the convergence point is directly through the paperclip. When the paperclip is located at your fusion point, begin to move it back and forth while holding the fusion point through the paperclip. If you move the clip slowly, your brain will begin to align your eyes so they point directly to what you want to see. This is a recalibration and your brain will begin to automatically fuse your vision perfectly.

Possible patterns you might see. Make sure that the center point is right through the paper cip.

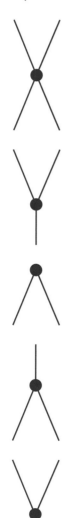

All the mind needs is a reference and it will automatically make the adjustments for you. Do this exercise for a few minutes only, but do it about ten times a day until you can easily place the center of the cross anywhere on the string. Look away and look back and still find the cross through the paperclip. Then you have completed the exercise and have perfect convergence. In my experience, which tallies with the findings, this adjustment takes place quite rapidly and is highly effective. Research suggests more than 85 percent efficacy.

Convergence and reading

I often come across people with presbyopia (the need for reading glasses) where convergence is a big part of the problem. For one reason or another, the eyes develop difficulty in turning inward. The outer eye muscle is held too tight. Perhaps it is because their mothers told them not to cross their eyes as a child. In fact, for proper reading your eyes need to turn in (converge) a few degrees. If not, your near point of clear vision will drift further and further away and you will develop presbyopia.

Convergence can be corrected optically with prism elements. A prism bends the light towards the base of the prism and thereby corrects for the divergence. The disadvantage of prism therapy is that they quickly become very heavy. Also there are limitations to the range of vision divergence a prism can compensate for. Prisms are mostly used for treating strabismus. Of course, the prism will do nothing for the underlying convergence problem.

Convergence practice exercise

This exercise is designed for developing perfect convergence. Take a string and measure off 2 meters. Next, tie knots every 10 cm along the string. To make the knots stand out you can paint them with colored markers. Alternatively you can tie on colourful beads or small plastic rings. Colored paperclips would also do.

To perform the exercise, tie one end of the string to a door handle or to the back of a chair. Take the free end of the string and put it on the tip of your nose. Keep the string straight and look down its length. You will see a cross centered over every knot you look at. Move your attention from knot to knot and notice how the cross keeps jumping. Vary the exercise, looking at every second knot, every third knot and so on. Also, look away and find the cross again instantly. Develop the ability to see the cross when you look up, down and to the side. Do this exercise about five times a day until you can do it effortlessly; then you will have perfect convergence.

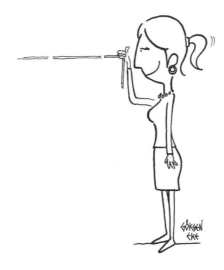

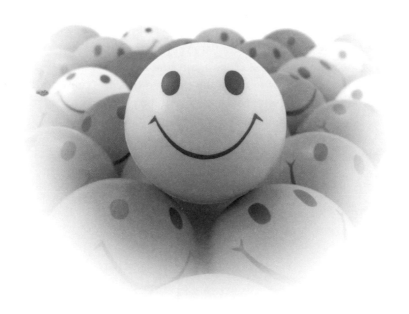

20. Strabismus

Strabismus is a condition where one eye is turned in a different direction from the eye that is used for seeing. The divergence can be towards the center and is then called esotropia (from the Greek *ese* meaning inward). The inner recti muscle is too tense causing the eye to be turned too far inward. This accounts for almost 50 percent of all cases. When the eye turns out it is known as exotropia (from the Greek *exo* meaning outward). The divergence may be only slight and almost imperceptible to very severe, in which case the pupil is almost hidden in the corner of the eye. The divergence may also occur upwards and is then called hyperphoria (from the Greek *hyper* meaning above) or it can be downwards and is then referred to as hypophoria (from the Greek *hypo* meaning down). Strabismus is usually present at a very early age but can also develop in adults.

Because of the divergent stressful double vision that is experienced, the brain switches off the image from the divergent eye creating amblyopia (or lazy eye). This is the reason strabismus and amblyopia are associated.

There is also a type of strabismus known as heterophoria, which is a deviation that is held in check by normal convergence. In some people you might notice a slight divergence, especially when they are engaged in internal processing. However, when they focus on you or some object of interest the eyes are perfectly co-ordinated.

The cause of strabismus is not known at the present time. The usual approach is to first treat amblyopia if it is present. Strabismus itself may be treated by inserting prisms into the glasses in order to correct for the divergence. However, there is a limit to how much divergence can be treated (up to 5D prism diopters) before the glasses become too heavy. Fresnel lenses are sometimes used since they are lighter and can be constructed to correct a higher degree of divergence.

Correcting the divergence with optics does very little to address the underlying causes. The angle of the prism shifts the image position so the brain perceives it to be within the range of convergence. But the moment you remove the prism you still have strabismus.

Surgery is another option that is often recommended by ophthalmologists since it corrects the eye position so the cosmetic appearance is improved. However, the vision is not always improved when surgically shortening or repositioning the eye muscle. In any case, surgery should only be contemplated after all other options have been exhausted.

Ophthalmologist William H. Bates (1920) concluded that strabismus was caused not by the strength of the muscles but by strain. In that respect he felt there was no difference between near-sight, far-sight and astigmatism. They were all functional problems that respond to Vision Training.

Strabismus is usually a condition that afflicts children. However, it is not unheard of in adults. In many cases the individual has been to see a profusion of doctors at various clinics. Often the traditional treatment procedures lead nowhere and only build more frustration for all concerned.

In my experience children respond very quickly to Vision Training and are greatly relieved when they don't have to wear eye-patches and undergo other uncomfortable treatments. One case involved a 9-year-old girl who had been to a number of eye doctors. She was wearing bifocal glasses at the time I saw her. Her distant vision was quite good but her problem was seeing medium and near objects. The doctors recommended surgery but the parents were reluctant to subject their daughter to this, especially when they realized that the chance of success was not very high.

First I taught her the butterfly exercise (see below), which is designed to train the wandering eye to work together with the normal eye. The girl responded very well because the next day she walked into the Vision Training class like a little princess. She had been without glasses for most of the day and she could now make her eyes converge on close objects and she could see the phantom cross on the string, which indicated that both eyes were working and converging towards the object she wanted to see. After a few more sessions her eyes were functioning normally and would only begin to diverge slightly if she was getting tired.

Another case involved a professional woman who had developed strabismus with the right eye moving out (exotropia). This happened shortly after she had to suddenly move house. It seemed that the stress had caused her eye to diverge. She had seen a number of eye doctors and they had all told her that surgery was the only way to correct her problem.

The woman had attended one of my Vision Training classes the previous year so she had some idea of what might be possible using natural approaches. However, she did not know exactly what to do.

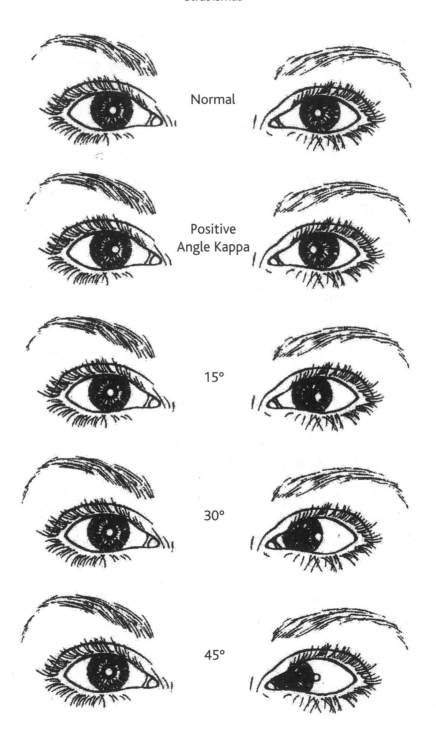

Normal

Positive
Angle Kappa

15°

30°

45°

Again I taught her the butterfly exercise designed to help co-ordinate the two eyes. Amazingly, after doing the exercise just a few times her eyes started to converge normally. This was a case where the divergence of the eye had not yet been firmly established. The human brain learns amazingly fast.

In most cases strabismus responds wonderfully to Vision Training. Obviously it is best to do the exercises with someone else, because you cannot see your own eyes and do the exercise at the same time.

How to test for strabismus

There are two simple tests you can make to determine the degree and type of strabismus by using a small penlight held at eye level from a distance. Shine the light into the eyes so you can see the light spot on the cornea. In normal eyes the spot will be right in the center of the black pupil. The more the eye diverges the higher the degree of strabismus.

Note that 1 mm displacement (called positive kappa if the eye turns in and negative kappa if the eye turns out) is considered normal.

The cross-over test is used to reveal the full extent of strabismus. The test uses an occluder (something that will cover the eye) and transfers it from eye to eye. The longer the occluder is held before transferring, the more disruptive it is to the fusion. This test is also done with a semi-transparent material to reveal if there is latent (hidden) strabismus. If latent strabismus is present then the eye affected will turn behind the occluder.

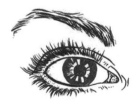 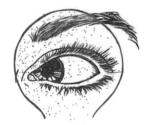

Vision Training principles for strabismus

We assume that strabismus is caused by poor co-ordination of the eye muscles. The object is to teach the brain to balance the muscles so the eyes will converge properly.

- Train the eye co-ordination in order to correct the divergence.

- Encourage the brain to use both eyes and get three-dimensional vision.

- Deal with the near-sight often present in the divergent eye.

In Vision Training we think of the exterior eye muscles as if they were a hydraulic system. Therefore, in strabismus we need to adjust the setting of the muscle that is held too tense and to firm up the muscle that is relaxed too much. In other words try to encourage a natural balance in the way the eyes are co-ordinated.

How well does Vision Training work for strabismus? Clara Hackett, in her book *Relax and See*, writes of her strabismus cases:

> There were 179 crossed eye students. 71 have achieved straight eyes and also have good fusion; 96 have straight eyes and good fusion except that there is a slight diversion from the norm when they are ill, emotionally upset or fatigued. 12 had no enduring improvement. (1955: 25)

This is a 90.5 percent success rate and is far better than what can be achieved with optical and medical methods. Children usually respond very quickly to Vision Training so the amount of time to be invested is usually only a few weeks and at the most a few months of daily training.

The wonderful thing about Vision Training is that the child is getting his or her normal vision restored. Clara Hackett's results, as noted above, are typical. In continental Europe the focus of functional optometrists is the treatment of strabismus in children. It is a program that lasts for about a year with regular visits to the optometrist and promises a very high degree of success.

There are two parts to the strabismus training:

- The first objective is to correct the divergence between the two eyes by encouraging flexibility in the eye muscles. We want to encourage the strabismic eye to co-ordinate with the other eye. This is done by using a piece of string as the reference point. The aim is to see the phantom cross that is present when the eyes are co-ordinated and converge on the object of interest.

● Secondly, we need to train the divergent eye, since it is usually more myopic than the dominant eye. In children this may be of lesser consequence, since the difference may be within the accommodative powers of the eye.

For the major part of strabismus training, we use a piece of string as a feedback device. In Vision Training it is important to always involve the brain to provide a clear response. The string provides both a measure of progress as well as clear feedback as to when you have succeeded.

The butterfly exercise

To attain the first objective of correcting the divergence between the two eyes, follow these steps. You will need somebody to assist with this exercise.

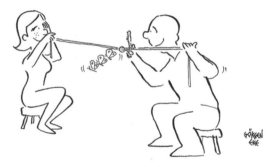

1. Hold the string to the tip of your nose in such a way that you have a straight line. Ask your assistant to hold the other end of the string.

2. Cover the good eye by placing a hand over it to block out all vision. This will force the brain to engage the divergent eye. Usually the eye is perfectly capable of moving and focusing on the object of interest.

3. Use a colorful object such as a marker pen and move the pen in the plane where the eye is diverging. For example, if the eyes are moving inward (esotropia) then move the pen back and forth so the brain moves the eye muscles that need to be adjusted. Move the pen back and forth (in the plane where the eye diverges) using larger and larger movements so that you become aware that your eyes can indeed track an object. Then make the movements smaller and smaller as you settle on the string, like a butterfly fluttering about before

finally settling on a flower. The gradually smaller movements help train the divergent eye.

4.   Now very slowly open the good eye. At one point you will have a brief glimpse of the phantom cross that occurs when both eyes converge. Initially this may be just a brief moment. Eventually it will be longer and longer until the eyes begin to track together.

5.   When the eyes begin to track together, you follow the marker pen with both eyes, training them to move in unison. This movement initially takes place in the same plane. When the eyes are comfortable tracking in one plane, begin to move the marker in and out so the eyes need to converge at different planes in order to follow it. You are then practicing the second objective of getting both eyes to co-ordinate in a natural way.

Do this exercise for just a few minutes at a time but frequently during the day, as is convenient. It is better to do the exercise ten times a day for 1 minute than to do 30 minutes of the exercise once. The objective is to train the mind to co-ordinate the eye muscles so both eyes converge on the object of interest.

With children it is best to use different objects in order to catch their attention. It is also very important to make the exercise a game and not insist upon doing it because it has to be done. Remember, the child's mind must be involved and this is best presented as entertainment. Perhaps you could give a little reward when certain milestones are achieved. This usually helps to keep the interest level high.

The long body swing exercise

This exercise has been used by vision trainers since the turn of the century and has been found particularly useful for strabismus. It is sometimes referred to as the elephant swing since the movement resembles the movement an elephant makes when chewing its food.

Swinging slowly from side to side relaxes the eyes and therefore encourages natural eye co-ordination. It works with the mind's natural tendency to converge on a desired object. As you slowly swing from side to side, the mind will naturally try to converge on the object of interest as you swing by. This exercise is best done with children old enough to understand the instructions.

1.   Stand with your feet parallel and sufficiently apart for comfortable balance. Shift your weight from one foot to the other in the easy swaying motion you

have seen elephants make in the zoo. As you sway gently from side to side let your head and shoulders turn with your swing. Let the arms and hands hang limply from loose shoulders allowing the momentum to lift and swing them as you turn from side to side. Count aloud rhythmically in tempo with the swing. This is important because when you are counting aloud or singing it is impossible to hold your breath. Deep rhythmic breathing is essential for relaxation and good vision.

2. Be sure that neck, shoulder and chest muscles are loose and relaxed. Swing all of your body to one side, then to the other. As you count from 1 to 60 you develop the relaxation you need. From 60 to 100, you fully release nerves and muscles. Best of all, your eyes begin to shift with their many involuntary vibrations, which brings improved vision. You are not able to sense this but you will know that it is taking place when the entire room starts slipping past you in the opposite direction as if you were traveling in a row of railway cars going back and forth. Perhaps you can find a piece of music that will help you to sway in time.

Do this exercise slowly. The objective is to relax. Should you feel dizzy, you are leaving your eyes behind. Be sure you get the feeling of motion as you swing. When mind and eyes allow the world to pass by without clinging and fixing on passing objects, carsickness, elevator sickness and seasickness will be a thing of the past.

Do this exercise two or three times a day to induce general relaxation and better eye co -ordination.

The mirror swing exercise

This exercise comes from Clara Hackett and is described in her book *Relax and See* (1955: 181). The purpose is the same as the full body swing – to relax the eyes and encourage them to track together. It is a convenient exercise to do in the morning whilst you are in the bathroom.

1. With feet slightly apart stand with your back to the mirror.

    If your left eye turns in, then cover your right eye with one hand and look straight ahead with your left eye.

2. Slowly turn the upper part of your body left until you see your left eye in the mirror. Slowly return to the start position. Do this four to six times.

3.   Next cover your left eye and turn right to see the right eye in the mirror. Do this two or three times.

The principle behind this exercise is to always encourage the diverging eye to straighten out. So start the turn in the direction in which you want the eye to turn. If the eye turns too much to the right, then you should turn towards the left.

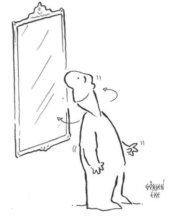

The balance swing exercise

This is another of Clara Hackett's exercises for strabismus. The purpose here, once again, is to encourage the eyes to track. It is always good to have a variety of exercises to play with.

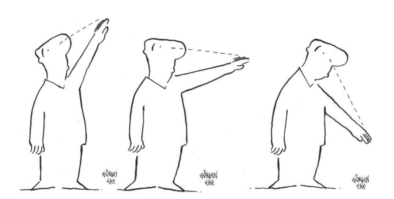

1.   Stand with your feet slightly apart and with both arms stretched out at shoulder level. Always turn to the opposite side from where the eye diverges. So if your left eye turns in, or your right eye turns out, you turn your head to the left.

2.   Bend the upper part of your body to the right, raising your left arm to the ceiling and at the same time lowering the right arm to the floor.

3.   Straighten, and then bend to the left, lowering the left arm and raising the right arm. Keep watching the left hand as your head and body move. Do this

six to eight times. Then turn and do the same thing while watching the right hand.

If your right eye turns in, or your left eye turns out, complete as above but start by turning your head towards your right hand.

Tromboning exercise

This exercise was originally suggested by Janet Goodrich in her excellent book *Natural Vision Improvement* (1986: 129). As the name suggests, you move an object back and forth just as a trombone player moves the slide on his instrument.

First you need to create your trombone. Make a paddle similar to a table tennis paddle from some colorful cardboard. Put some attention-grabbing stickers on the cardboard so that there are lots of interesting things to look at.

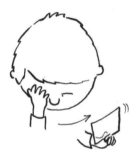

- If the right eye diverges out, then move the paddle across your body's midline and outwards to the left. Cover the left eye as you slowly move the paddle back and forth while looking at some of the details in the stickers and trying to keep them in focus for as long as possible.

If the eye turns in then move the cardboard from the nose and out.

- If the left eye diverges out, then move the paddle across your body's midline and outwards to the right. Cover the right eye as you slowly move the paddle back and forth while looking at some of the details in the stickers and trying to keep them in focus for as long as possible.

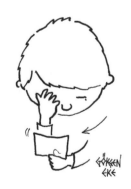

- If the left eye goes in, then move the paddle away from your body's midline to the left. Cover the right eye as you move the paddle from the center and out, while looking at the stickers and trying to keep them in focus for as long as possible.

- If the right eye goes in, then move the paddle away from your body's midline to the right. Cover the left eye as you move the paddle from

If the eye turns then move the cardboard from outside towards the nose.

the center and out, while looking at the stickers and trying to keep them in focus for as long as possible.

This exercise can be done with almost any prop – whenever is convenient. The movement encourages the mind to adjust the co-ordination of the eye muscles. Repeat this exercise for short periods of time, but do it frequently.

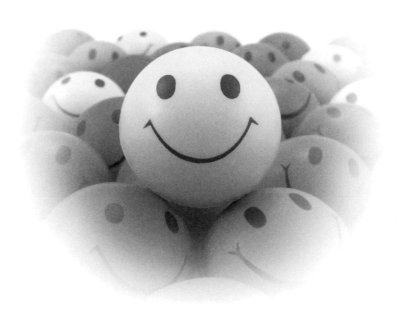

21. Amblyopia

Amblyopia is defined as defective visual acuity which persists after correction of the refraction error and removal of any pathological obstacle to vision. This is a condition of unknown origin where vision in one eye is switched off by the brain. Recently amblyopia has been thought of as a sensory adaptation to strabismus, a condition where one eye looks out in the wrong direction.

Some clinicians believe that there is a sensitive period of development for various visual functions. Experiments made with monkeys suggest that early visual deprivation (age 3 to 6 months) abolishes pattern and binocular vision. A later onset of visual deprivation (up to 25 months) results in reduced contrast sensitivity. Vaegan and Taylor (1980) note that visual deprivation in the first three years of life left only rudimentary vision. Patients with a later onset of vision deprivation suffered less visual loss, and patients deprived after ten years of age suffered no loss. Incidentally, many of the patients in the study showed substantial improvements in vision after optical correction and Vision Training (orthoptic treatment).

Amblyopia may develop due to a number of reasons such as:

- Deviating eye – Amblyopia is likely to develop in children under the age of 3 if one eye is deviating (turning in or out) as in strabismus. In untreated conditions a marked decrease in visual acuity may develop within just a few weeks.

- Defocused eye – When one eye is severely near-sighted and the images appear blurred at all distances (more than 4 diopters), amblyopia is likely to develop. Adults with one eye that is severely myopic may develop amblyopia if Vision Training is not undertaken, even if they wear corrective lenses.

- Deprived eye – Amblyopia can develop as a result of covering one eye for a whole day, for as little as a week, during the early stages of an infant's visual development.

The medical treatment of choice is patching the good eye, which over the years has been supplemented with active stimulation of the eye using electrical and chemical stimulants. Strategies used include total occlusion, excluding all light and form, such as using adhesive occludes worn on the skin. Opaque black contact lenses, frosted glass and other filters are also used to this end.

Amblyopia is treated in childhood and rarely starts after the age of 8. If strabismus is involved, surgical replacement of the eye muscles is often performed in an attempt to straighten the eye so that both eyes track together. This results in a more pleasing appearance.

The success rate with patches is not especially high. A study, conducted by Watson et al. (1985) compared the effects of full-time and part-time occlusion. It was found that 23 percent of the patients studied showed no improvement despite adequate and vigorous treatment. The argument that is often proffered to explain the failure of the method is that the patient is not following the instructions. However, this study was done in a hospital setting so there was no possibility of patients not following the regime.

People who have gone though this treatment in childhood will often tell you that they hated wearing the patch and that it didn't make much difference anyway.

If you are a parent you will know that it is virtually impossible to get a patch to stay on a child. Because of this, in some cases the children's elbows were actually put into splints to prevent them from ripping the patch off. I believe that today many people would consider this to be child abuse.

Recently I worked with a 7-year-old called Shara in Mexico. She'd had the lens removed from her left eye. The operation was successful but she had developed severe amblyopia in the eye. The eye looked lifeless and was beginning to divert slightly. Shara had not responded to any medical treatments. In essence, she had given up hope of ever regaining sight in her left eye.

Initially Shara did not respond to any of the exercises. She had perfect 20/20 vision in the right eye and was consequently using that eye all the time. The other children in the workshop were doing an exercise using eye-charts. In a moment of inspiration, I took down one of the charts and asked her to look at the large "E" about 20 cm from her left eye. She could recognize the "E." I asked her to relax her eyes by palming. Soon she was able to see the 20/200 and even the 20/160 line from 20 cm. This was a tremendous experience for both her and her mother because it now became apparent that her eye could respond to Vision Training.

The next day, after many short exercises, Shara was able to see even smaller letters with her left eye. Most important, however, was the changing appearance of her eye.

It had more life and was beginning to track together with the dominant right eye. Shara, with the help of her mother, needs to do exercises for a long time – perhaps years. The good news is that Shara now believes it is possible for her to get her vision back. After all, cataract removal does not affect the part of the eye that actually sees (i.e., the retina).

The problem with the traditional approach is that it is passive and does not involve the mind. You are, in essence, trying to use force to get the eyes to function normally.

Vision Training principles for amblyopia

- First establish the extent of vision in the amblyopic eye. This is done using a string and markers (see page 124).

- Train the amblyopic eye to see clearly inch by inch gradually extending the visual acuity.

The first milestone will be when you have reached the same near point for both eyes. The next milestone will be when you can manage to read using both eyes.

Include strabismus training, if necessary, to get both eyes to track together.

The Vision Training approach involves including the mind in the training. We assume that the eye has the capacity to see naturally, so it is just a matter of doing the right exercises with it. In many cases, involvement of cross-lateral movements, such as Brain Gym® exercises, are of great help in activating the various brain functions involved in well co-ordinated behaviour. Kids love to move around so Brain Gym exercises serve a useful function in making the session enjoyable and fun. It may take a long time and the exercises have to be done many times every day. However, there is a worthwhile reward – clarity of vision.

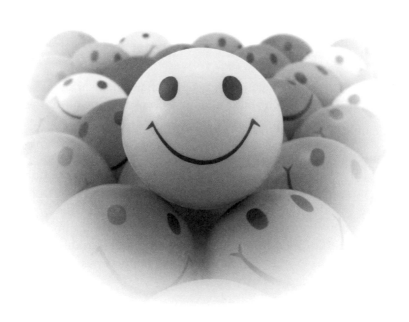

22. Color Perception

The Vision Training approach to color perception deficiency in the common red–green spectrum is to encourage finer differentiation of the problem colors. The instruction consists of exercises using colors, thus gaining a deeper understanding of how color works. Our ability to perceive colors is one of the things that makes the world beautiful. Colors are not only beautiful, they are also exceptionally useful. The color of an apple lets you know whether or not it is ripe. Colourful displays, book and magazine covers attract our attention. Colors are also essential to fashion. Each season has a new set of colors.

Color perception deficiency affects almost 8 percent of the male population. It is believed to be inherited, usually from the maternal grandfather. The typical red–green color perception deficiency can be greatly improved by Vision Training.

The scientific study of color starts with Iasaac Newton's great work, *Opticks* (1704). This is an extraordinary work detailing Newton's experiments in Trinity College, Cambridge. In *Opticks*. Newton showed that white light is made up of all the spectral colors. The later wave theory of light made it clear that each color corresponds to a specific frequency.

In the nineteenth century Thomas Young proposed the trichromatic color theory which suggests that there are three primary colors. German scientist Hermann von Helmholtz developed Young's ideas further and it became the Young–Helmholtz theory. There are three color sensitive receptors (cone cells) which respectively respond to red, green and blue. All colors are seen by a mixture of signals from the three color receptors. Incidentally, this is the same principle behind your computer screen. In computer parlance it is known as the RBG color system.

Opponent color theory

German physiologist Ewald Hering noted that red and green are never seen simultaneously and the color red/green is never used. Colors are either red or green, but not both. The same is true for blue and yellow. This observation led Hering to propose the opponent color vision theory (1964).

In the late 1950s Leo Hurvich and Dorothea Jameson provided quantitative data in support of the notion that color opponency plays an important role in processing color information. They used a hue cancellation procedure (hue is added to the stimulus until it turns white) to determine spectral sensitivities of the red–green and blue–yellow opponent channels.

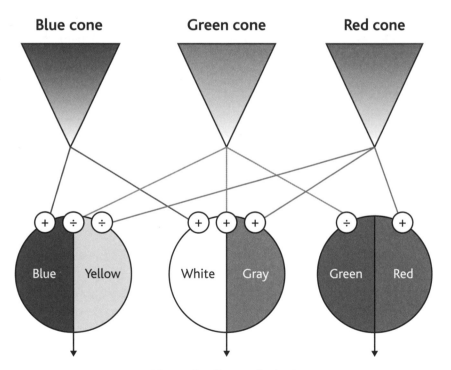

Nerves leading to the brain

It is believed that the red–green and blue–yellow channels only code hue information. An independent brightness channel presumably codes the brightness. If the frequency of action potential is plotted as a function of wavelength then we see that a low wavelength stimulus (below 550 nm) causes inhibition, or a decreased firing rate from this cell. In contrast, a long-wavelength stimulus (longer than 550 nm) produces excitation, or an increased rate of neural firing. When a photosensitive cell responds to one portion of the spectrum with excitation and another portion with inhibition, it is referred to as a color opponent neuron.

The discovery of color opponent neurons in the visual system tells us that the receptoral information (trichomacy) is coded in an opponent fashion at post-receptoral levels. In other words, the three classes of color sensitive cone cells are "wired" together in such a way that they are spectrally antagonistic. This opponent processing occurs very early in the visual system, at the level of horizontal cells. It is scientifically established that hue information is encoded by red–green and blue–yellow neurons which are also involved in the red–green color perception deficiency. It is not clear whether brightness information is encoded by these neurons or by a separate class of non-color opponent cells.

Hue discrimination

The hue defines the smallest wavelength of light with the smallest difference that it is possible to differentiate with the human eye. We notice that there is a dramatic increase in the red–green sensitivity, producing exceptional hue discrimination ability in the green–yellow–orange–red region. This is a very useful feature because various foods and fruits display their readiness to be eaten by their color change. You can instantly see whether or not a strawberry is ripe by its color.

Color film is a complex arrangement of the three primary color filters. Kodachrome slides are able to reproduce all the complexity of color seen in nature.

Color vision is very complex and cannot be reduced to simple theories. It depends not only on wavelengths and intensities, but also on differences in intensity between regions and whether the patterns are accepted as representing known objects. This involves high level processing in the brain which is extremely difficult to investigate.

The eye tends to accept white not as a particular mixture of colors, but rather the general illumination. Thus you see a car's headlights as white while on a country drive, but in town where there are bright white lights for comparison, they look quite yellow, and the same is true of candlelight. This means that what you take as a reference for white can shift. Expectation and knowledge of normal color is an important factor in color perception.

Color perception deficiency

Surprisingly, the common confusion of red with green was not discovered before the late eighteenth century, when chemist John Dalton found that he could not distinguish certain substances by their color although others could do so easily. Color vision tests depend on being able to isolate color as the sole identifying characteristic. Once this is established, it is easy to show whether a person has normal ability to distinguish between colors, or whether he or she sees as a single color that which others perceive as different colors. It is much more common to find a reduced sensitivity to certain colors than a complete absence of color.

The properties of red and green light required to match a monochromatic yellow is the most important measure of color deficiency. Lord Rayleigh discovered in 1881 that people who confuse red with green require a greater intensity of either red or green to match yellow. A special instrument, called an anomaloscope, has been developed for testing this color deficiency. The instrument takes advantage of the fact that yellow is always seen as a mixture of red and green.

The reason for red–green color perception deficiencies is not clear. However, experiments with the anomaloscope show that color anomaly cannot be due to color adaptation. The general belief is that red–green color perception deficiency is due to a reduction in the sensitivity of one or more color receptors (cone cells) in the retina, perhaps through partial loss of photo-pigment. There may be many causes, but it is not due to shortage of photo-pigment, otherwise the anomaloscope would not work. The common red–green color perception deficiency is more likely to be an interpretation of sensory data provided to the visual cortex that processes color vision.

The typical test used for defective red–green color perception is the Ishihara Color Test. This consists of scattered dots of different colors where the hues that are difficult for red–green deficiency people to see are used to form numbers. If these images are scanned into graphic software and the hue variable changed by about +70, a red–green color deficient person will clearly see the obscured numbers. Indeed, it may be possible to train the eye to see the colors that were confusing and then notice how they begin to be more distinct with less hue distortion.

The ability to label colors is, to a certain extent, a learned ability. As we grow up we learn to identify colors in the same way that we learn to recognize time on a watch. For some this learning is not quite complete, so color perception training may be necessary in order to improve the situation.

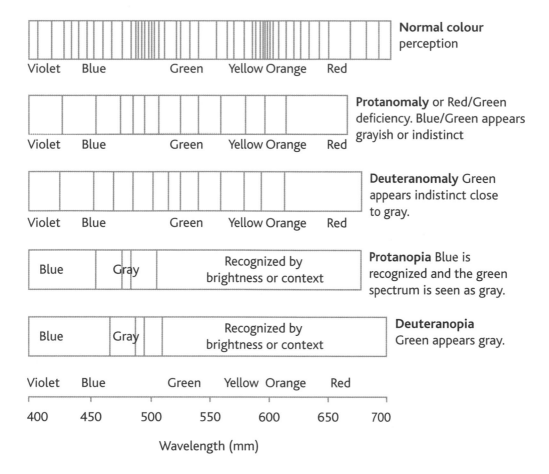

The graph above shows how people with normal color perception label colors. Each vertical bar indicates a successful identification. You will notice that there are many lines between blue and green and between yellow and orange. The blue–green spectrum is the one that causes the most trouble for people with the typical red–green color perception deficiency. Turquoise colors are confused with gray, especially if the intensity of the color is the same.

The other end of the spectrum also causes problems. Red-violet or scarlet colors are often confused with brown. As you can see, those with protanomaly and deuteranomaly can distinguish all the colors but with fewer distinctions between them.

It is possible to improve this discrimination by training your color perception and practicing the labeling skills. Most color perception deficiency is a red–green problem. This type of color vision is one of two main types related to the wavelength of the light. Long-wavelength red light (protanomaly) may be complete protanopia where blue is recognized but the green spectrum is perceived as white or gray and anything between green and red is distinguished by brightness or context. Each area appears to those with protanopia as one system of color with different brightness and saturation within each area.

With the more common protanomaly most colors are recognized. The part of the spectrum that normally appears blue-green is perceived by the person with protanomaly as a grayish or indistinct color. The complement to blue-green, which is red-violet, will also appear indistinct.

Middle wavelength green light may be complete deuteranopia where the part of the spectrum that is normally perceived as green, appears gray. The complementary color to green – violet-red – also appears gray or indistinct.

The less severe deficiency is deuteranomaly. In this case, there is no part of the spectrum that appears to be gray, but the green part of the spectrum (which appears to the deuteranope as gray) appears indistinct and close to gray.

Protanomaly and deuteranomaly are easier to improve than the more severe protanopia and deuteranopia. The latter have fewer distinctions to begin with so there is much more work involved.

Counting colors

Some people have difficulty in distinguishing variations of a color. This exercise develops your ability to see and label colors in different materials and in different lights.

1. For a period of a day, start counting all the examples of a color you already know. For example, one of the primary colors, red, blue or yellow.

2. The next day count all the different shades of green you can find.

3. On another day count all the examples of other secondary colors you can find (the secondary colors are orange, green and violet).

4. Next, begin to identify and count all the gray shades you can find.

5. Progress to browns and earth colors like ochre, sienna and burnt umber.

Notice what the colors look like in different lights. How does brown look in the morning compared to how it looks at sunset? How does it look on a rainy day? Counting and identifying colors develops and refines your ability to see them. A large part of color perception difficulty has to do with the number of colors you can distinguish. Developing more reference experiences with progressively finer hue distinctions will eventually lead to better color perception.

Matching colors

When you develop your ability to distinguish more colors with the working with colors exercise below then you can begin to match colors. Perhaps you can even begin to learn more about the different ways of organizing colors.

1. Practice naming colors and have a friend verify them for you. You need feed-back to keep your progress on the right track.

2. Arrange colors in order of intensity, so you have the lighter shade at one end and getting progressively darker and darker. Try to make the difference in hue as small as possible. Play especially with the blue-green and red-violet colors, as they are the ones you are likely to have the most difficulty distinguishing.

3. Progress to matching different materials and arrange them in order of inten-sity and hue. Try working with pieces of cloth and match sewing threads to the colors of the cloth.

Be creative and match and order things. The more you play this game the better.

Working with colors

In order to build broader color distinction, it is very valuable to experiment with either watercolors or pastels. The objective is to understand how colors work and especially what they look like. Color pigments behave differently according to the light, but in practice you are mostly asked to recognize the colors reflected off printed cards.

Play with the primary colors

All possible variations of color can be mixed from just the three primary colors – red, yellow and blue – so the first step is to play with these colors. Find the brightest yellow possible. It is probably called something like chromium yellow or bright yellow. Paint samples on a piece of white paper. Experiment with different intensities of yellow from 100 percent to just 1 percent – a very pale yellow that is almost imperceptible. Now look at these color samples in different lights and notice how they change.

Try painting the same yellow on neutral gray paper and notice how the colors change compared to the same color on a white background. When you are using pastels, try painting different intensities of yellow on black or brown paper. Notice how this changes the appearance of the colors. Next try to find similarities between all the test colors you have made so far.

Do the same with the blue and red paints. Some of the colors will be easy for you to notice, while others might be a stretch. In either case you are enriching your sense of color.

Play with the secondary colors

The secondary colors are made from mixing equal amounts of the three primary colors. First mix red and yellow to produce a bright orange. Next mix yellow and blue to produce green. Finally mix red and blue to produce violet. You now have samples of the three secondary colors and can make a six color spectrum. Take each of the 12 colors and make different densities of each of them. Notice what they look like.

The next project is to add one more color on each side of the six colors you already have. This will give you a 12 color circle. You can now begin to see how the colors blend together. If you like, you can add one more color between each of the 12 colors you have already. This will show an even finer blend between the colors.

Playing with gray and black

Next make a series of samples of gray and black, so you can get an idea of how black pigment behaves. Notice that pigments may look different depending on their purity. Begin to match gray shades and colored shades according to their intensity.

Playing with brown and earth colors

Browns are pigment mixtures of orange and black. Try mixing orange and black in equal quantities and then make this color into a series of lighter and lighter shades. Play with burnt umber, sienna, burnt sienna and ochre. Notice the different intensities and compare and match brown shades with the other color samples you have in your collection.

Experiment with adding slight amounts of violet and red to the browns and notice how this affects the colors. By now you already have a good understanding of how colors appear and how they work together. You could also read about how colors have been organized into different color systems to help you further.

Blending colors

The problematic area for you is likely to be in identifying the blends that lie between blue and green. This is the most difficult area for protanomaly eyes. To develop your ability to identify these colors, take an A3 sheet of paper and draw a large box filling most of the paper. Next divide this box into 10 levels from top to bottom. Then make 10 vertical columns so you end up with a grid of 100 squares.

Label the upper right hand corner 0 percent and the next lower box 10 percent, 20 percent and so on. Do the same horizontally. You will end up with a sheet that has progressive intensity from the right corner to the left corner and from top to bottom.

Next make a gradation of gray along the side. This will serve as a comparison of intensity. Now fill in the colors column by column. You will end up with a color chart that shows the gradual blend of green and blue. The diagonal from right top to left bottom includes all the colors you need to practice identifying.

Make another chart using red and violet. This is the complementary color of blue-green, another area where you need to develop finer hue distinction.

Arranging colors

Here is another exercise that is useful for arranging color samples in order of intensity. This exercise will develop your ability to label colors correctly. Initially you may need help from someone with good color perception to verify your arrangement.

Cut out samples of the colors you have made during the previous exercises. Alternatively you could use a collection of paint swatches. The purpose of this exercise is to arrange samples according to their intensity. Pay special attention to colors that have the same intensity, but a different hue. You are extending the limits of your ability to distinguish colors.

Now you can progress to matching and arranging different kinds of material. These could be fabric samples, pieces of thread and so on. Matching sewing thread to the color of fabrics is a great way of training your color perception. It is a game you can play whenever you like.

23. The Visually Impaired

Visual impairment varies a great deal with some individuals having absolutely no visual stimulus whatsoever. However, many people who are considered legally blind actually have some light perception and can benefit from Vision Training exercises. Many of those who have some quality of light perception – that is they can distinguish day and night and can recognize bright light – can improve their vision and possibly achieve object recognition. Clara Hackett, a Vision Trainer working during the 1940s and 1950s, reported that of the eight people she worked with that had only light perception, one man was able to resume his regular work and four attained object perception. Only three of the people she worked with showed no improvement (Hackett, 1955: 7).

People with object perception – who can identify pieces of furniture or people moving about – can often attain improvement of vision ability. Hackett reported that of 14 people with some object perception, eight gained useful vision and were no longer considered "blindish." Of the 34 people who were considered occupationally blind, 16 were able to work again, while eight others showed improvement in visual acuity. Ten had no appreciable improvement.

This is wonderful news; at least there is the possibility of improvement. The possibly traumatic events that lead to a diagnosis of visual impairment can leave a person without hope. While there is no guarantee that Vision Training exercises will work, there is the possibility that vision can stabilize and even improve. Whatever degree of vision you have now, why not try the following techniques for a month? If after a month you are not sure if you are really improving or only imagining it, continue for another month, and by that time you will have no doubts. It will be clear by then whether or not there are signs of definite improvement.

Gaining light perception

If you have no light perception at all, then your first efforts should be directed towards achieving this. The techniques are very simple. When the sun shines, turn your closed eyelids towards the sun for a minute or two about ten times a day. When you turn your head towards the sun you will feel its warmth. Move your head slowly from side to side always keeping your closed eyes towards the sun. The energy from the sun is pure and will help to energize your eyes. It is safe as long as you keep your eyes closed.

Relaxing your eyes

Relaxation is an important aspect of your Vision Training. To palm your eyes, rub your hands together vigorously so that they get warm. Place the palms of your hands over your closed eyelids without touching the eyes, with your fingers folded over your forehead. While palming try to imagine what it would be like to actually see some light. Think about things you remember with pleasure. Visualization is known to activate the mind–body connection. The basic principle is that energy follows thought, so the more things you can imagine the better.

Mapping across your senses

Your kinesthetic sense is highly developed and is used to discern where you are in space. Your hands, and especially your fingertips, are very sensitive to energy. With your hands you can learn to detect the energy emanating from people and objects. For example, most people can detect the energy radiated by different colors. Make index card size samples of bright primary colors (red, blue and yellow) and secondary colors (orange, green and violet) as well as black and white.

First test how black feels by letting your hand, either left or right, float over the paper. Sense what black feels like. Now sense the white and notice the difference. Go through the colors and get a sense of each one. To test your ability to sense the colors, mix up the cards and reverse them so the white side is up. Now try to find each color by feeling. If you have recollections of what those colors look like, then add the color to the impression.

Gaining object recognition

Start with something very simple, such as trying to distinguish two fingers against the light. Go on from there and explore the extent of your vision. How far to the right can you see? How far down can you see your fingers? This may take a long time so make it a game you can play every day. Eventually you may be able to see the five fingers of your hand at arm's length against the light.

The energy exercise on page 121, as well as sunning your eyes, helps create plenty of energy. Keep up the good work and you will develop object recognition to the fullest extent that is possible for you. This may be the ability to see large objects such as cars and houses, or it may be the ability to move around freely and be able to function as someone who is merely near-sighted.

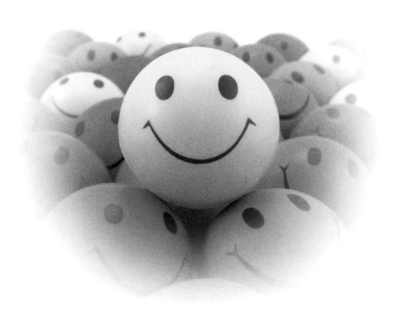

24. Beyond 20/20 Vision

During archery practice, officers found that the eyesight of their commandos appeared to improve when following the path of the arrow with their eyes in a state of relaxation. This technique not only improves focus, but stretches sharp vision to normal and beyond.

You can make improvements to your eyesight even if you already have excellent vision. I remember a workshop in Istanbul where there were a number of people who had naturally good eyesight. They attended my workshop because they wanted to keep it that way. We had a splendid view over the Bosphorus, so I suggested we play around with our visual abilities. There is a technique you can use to push vision beyond 20/20. First look at something further away than you actually need to see. In this case we used the buildings on the Asian side of the Bosphorus. Next look at something closer up. You will find that your eyes will then find it easier to focus on the nearer object.

This effect is enhanced if you do some swinging along the features of the distant object. Your eyes will follow your intention. If you send your attention out beyond what you can normally see, you are exercising and extending your visual capability.

Rescue teams flying over wilderness areas attempting to spot people lost or in distress use an imaginary grid as they focus on progressively smaller and smaller objects. The spotters with the best track record all have similar strategies.

During the First World War, the men who flew fighter planes did not have instruments to guide them so had to rely on good eyesight. The most successful pilots deliberately sent their eyes 10 kilometers out into the sky. The eyes will naturally settle a few hundred meters into space if you do not send your attention further out. The same goes for driving a car. Send your eyes out to the horizon, to the road far ahead, to the car in front of you and so on. Let your eyes roam the landscape. You will discover that your vision is improving.

Hunters are another group of people who naturally have great vision strategies. A hunter will scan the land ahead and notice things that are a little bit different, such as a few leaves on a tree that do not move in the right way because a deer is hiding there. Many hunters say they are looking for things that aren't there. Their minds are automatically attracted to things that are different, and their eyes will go to that point and instantly focus on a minute detail. It is a chunking down process where you notice a tree, then a particular branch, then a cluster of leaves and finally just one leaf or even the tip of a leaf. During this chunking down process your eyes will automatically follow your attention. In other words, your mind controls where your eyes will travel.

Another way of practicing your distance vision is to use the technique of looking at something that is further away than what you actually wish to see. Your eyes will attempt to focus on that distant object. When you look back at the object you wanted to see, you will notice that your eyes find it much easier to make it out. Experiment with this as you are driving. Look at road signs that are far away in the distance and then at ones that are closer and you will probably find that your vision begins to travel out much further than before. Like the First World War fighter pilots who deliberately sent their eyes 10 kilometers out into the sky, your eyes will also respond to the same strategy and begin to see things in the far distance.

If you would like to develop eagle eyes, play around with some of the ideas I have touched upon here. Make it a game which you can play all the time, whether you are walking, driving or simply relaxing.

Exercise to improve distance vision

Prepare for this exercise by palming for a few minutes.

1.   Take an eye-chart or a magazine with different sizes of text and place it in good daylight at eye level. Take a standing position far enough away from the chart so the letters are separate but not clear.

2.   Start a long swing past the chart, moving the head and body far to one side, then far to the other side, whilst not looking at anything in particular. The chart or magazine will seem to move by as you pass first one way and then the other.

3.   Keep swinging and shorten your swing from 50 cm on one side of the chart to 50 cm on the other side. Let the top of the chart pass just below your line of

vision so that you are not actually looking at it. If you have difficulty imagining this motion, close your eyes for a moment as you swing and the motion will come more easily.

4. Shorten the swing to 25 cm on each side of the chart, then to 15 cm, then to 5 cm, always keeping the top edge in rhythmic motion from side to side. Remember to breathe throughout this exercise and do a few rest swings with closed eyes now and then, imagining the motion as you swing.

5. When the chart has minimum motion from side to side, take a deep breath and flash all the way down the letters. They will be clear.

Practice this exercise for 5 minutes a few times every day as you move further and further away from the chart on your way to perfect vision.

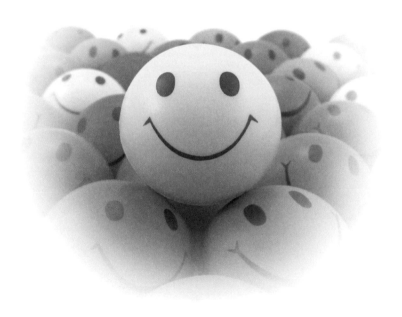

25. Mono-Vision

Having mono-vision means that you are using one eye for near tasks like reading and the other eye for tasks that involve seeing at a distance. With this arrangement, it would appear that your vision is entirely normal. However, it is at the expense of three-dimensional perception. Mono-vision is not advantageous, for instance, in the field of sport, where you may need to catch a ball or judge distance. In some cases people get fitted with two different lenses or have laser treatment that results in mono-vision.

Using one eye for reading and the other for driving is not a natural or desirable state of affairs. In Vision Training we always recommend that people work towards equalizing their eyes to give them more similar visual acuity. In the case of people with asymmetric visual perception, they have a condition known as anisometropia.

To equalize visual perception, first start by working to bring in the near point, so that both eyes can read small print from a distance of 15 cm. This is normal near-point acuity. When this is accomplished, both of your eyes will be involved in the reading process. Be sure to also check eye co-ordination (i.e., the cross on the string). This will take a bit of effort, as initially your brain may be so accustomed to switching eyes that it will continue in its habit of using the eyes one at a time. The second objective is to increase the distance vision of the weaker eye. The procedure will be the same as for a highly myopic eye. Keep working with each eye until their visual acuity is the same and then work with both eyes until you have perfect vision. The challenge here is to keep motivating yourself to do the exercises, as most of the time your eyes seem to operate normally just as they are. However, the fact remains that something in this visual system could go out of balance, in which case it is likely that you will experience problems. So it is best to start these exercises while they are relatively easy to do.

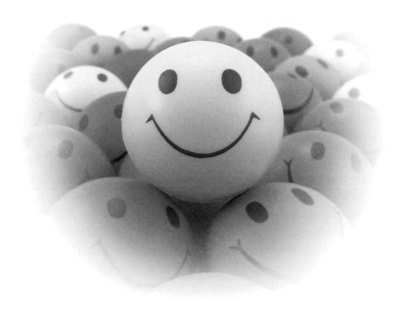

26. Sunglasses

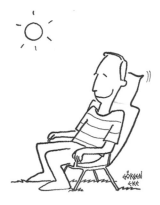

How did the phenomenon of sunglasses originate? Was it born out of advances in technology and the invention of versatile plastic? Or was it a mere fashion trend? Supposedly the reason we wear sunglasses is to protect ourselves from exposure to ultraviolet rays. In recent years ultraviolet light has come to be seen as something wrought with danger. However, the fact is that mankind has evolved over hundreds of thousands of years without the benefit of sunglasses. Research shows that the simple act of wearing a hat can cut UV exposure by 34 percent.

During the 1920s and 1930s sunlight, including the ultraviolet spectrum, was successfully used to treat such conditions as tuberculosis, rheumatoid arthritis, eczema, herpes, asthma and other health problems.

The 1903 Nobel Prize in medicine went to Niels Finsen of Denmark for developing the successful treatment of skin tuberculosis using ultraviolet light. Finsen also used light for other skin problems, for example, red light to prevent scar formation from smallpox.

Ultraviolet rays are the spectrum just below visible light and are divided into three bands.

High energy ultraviolet is called UV-C and is in the range of 100–290 ηm. This is generally only encountered in special situations such as arc welding or germicidal sterilization lamps. Since the cornea absorbs nearly all radiation below 290 ηm, protective gear such as welding masks or enclosed sterilization units are essential. Avoid looking into this light – it is dangerous.

Medium energy ultraviolet is called UV-B and is in the range of 290–320 ηm. The cornea absorbs most of this range and the lens take up the rest – only 1 percent reaches the retina. UV-B causes sunburn. However, it also activates the vital synthesis of vitamin D and the absorption of calcium and other minerals. Research shows that UV-B may also be a factor in the formation of cortical cataracts.

Low energy ultraviolet is called UV-A and is in the range of 320–380 ηm. This band is responsible for your suntan and photosensitive reactions which initiate the oxidative process associated with free radicals and the formation of cataracts. The lens absorbs more than half the UV-A rays that enter the eye.

It is important to be aware that any kind of light, not just UV light, will initiate a photosensitive reaction in the eye. To prevent this from occurring you would have to live in total darkness. It makes a lot more sense to combat this damage by taking vitamin C supplements. Exposure to ultraviolet light is essential for the body to be able to function.

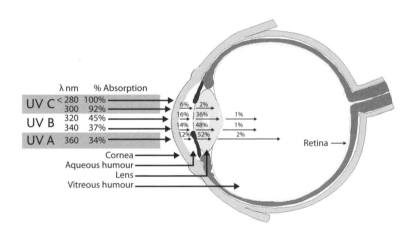

Wearing sunglasses can be appropriate if you are in an environment where there is very strong sunlight. For example, fresh snow reflects about 80 percent of UV light; consequently sunglasses are apposite accessories for winter sports.

The amount of UV light that reaches the eye depends on the season and the environment. For example, over 90 percent of incident UV light penetrates cloud cover and 95 percent of incident UV penetrates water – 50 percent down to a depth of 2 meters – so snorkeling on a cloudy day will still give you a suntan.

Sunglasses could also be appropriate if you go on vacation to a different part of the world. For example, if you travel from London to Jamaica, you should take your shades with you, as your eyes are not used to either the intensity of light or the ultraviolet rays on a typical sunny day in the Caribbean. If you are traveling in the other direction, however, don't bother with sunglasses, as the northern sun is not strong enough to be an issue.

If you wear sunglasses all the time then you are inadvertently training your eyes to be over-sensitive to the light. You may have experienced this if you have worn lenses that automatically change according to the intensity of the light. Many people find that when they remove these lenses, the light makes their eyes hurt. Getting progressively stronger and stronger prescription sunglasses is working at cross purposes.

Remember that your eyes are designed for light, so artificially filtering it out interferes with nature's design. People wearing dark sunglasses for prolonged periods of time tend to develop a sensitivity to light, similar to that experienced after working indoors all day and then suddenly walking out into bright sunlight. The light will hurt your eyes until they adjust. This is a natural adjustment process.

I remember a woman in one of my workshops in Vancouver who told me that she wore her sunglasses in the swimming pool to protect her eyes against the UV rays. She wanted to know what she could do about light sensitivity. The scientific name for this is photopia.

There is a very simple way to train your eyes to be comfortable in bright light. Simply let the sun shine on your closed eyelids for a few seconds. This will gradually train your eyes to adjust to brighter light. It's that simple – and it's effective. After all, the sun is the source of life.

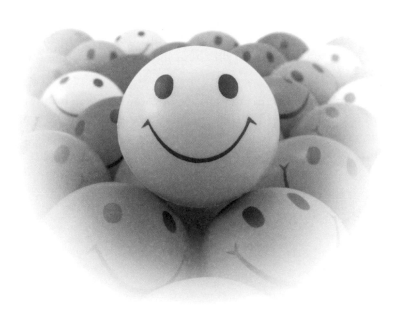

27. Surgical Eyes

In recent years there has been much publicity and enticing advertising extolling an amazingly simple surgical procedure that can restore your vision to perfect. This is a prime example of an easy fix. The invitation is to have your eyes corrected for good in a procedure that takes just a few minutes. I have even seen laser clinics provide a free video recording of your operation and in some cases the surgery is even performed in your local shopping mall!

Structure of the cornea

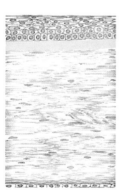

Pavement epithelium
5 or 6 layers thick
Bowman's layer

Stroma

Descement's membrane
Endothelium

Any incision in corneal tissues that damages the Bowman's layer will induce permanent change in corneal curvature. The thickness of the cornea is about 0.5 mm.

Usually this procedure is presented as simple, safe and painless. While there are many who have benefited from this operation, there are also plenty of people who have had their vision ruined for life. There can be quite a lot of pain in the days following the surgery. More than half of the superficial nerve fibers in the cornea are severed with the popular LASIK procedure. This impacts on the natural blink rate, which slows down causing the eyes to become dry. Patients often have to use eye drops for months before their eyes go back to normal.

Remember that the cornea is only about half a millimeter thick so any surgery performed has to be highly precise. Also, since there are no blood vessels in the cornea, healing takes many months. Some researchers say that the flap which is cut during the LASIK procedure never fully heals. In addition, corneal tissue is removed by the laser and as a consequence between 30 and 40 percent of corneal strength is lost, never to be regained. Cases are now emerging where the cornea bulges out, leading to a condition called keratoconus, which causes the eye to become pointed in shape. In some cases a corneal transplant may need to be performed in order to save the vision in the affected eye.

The law in the U.S. specifies that an M.D. must perform laser surgery but there is no specific training requirement. Any M.D., even a gynecologist or a pediatrician, can attend a weekend seminar put on by the laser manufacturer and legally start performing refractive surgery the following Monday. The drawbacks associated with this bonanza range from hard sell methods to an assortment of books about laser surgery that the doctor who performs your operation can distribute with his name inserted on the flyleaf as the author. You can even win free laser surgery as a prize in competitions. In the rush to make money, doctors and clinics sometimes conveniently forget to mention potential problems or to screen patients carefully before the procedure. The doctors consider the operation to have been a success if the patient can subsequently clearly see the 20/20 line on the eye-chart. However, it is possible to be able to have 20/20 vision but acquire other problems such as loss of low light vision, which can spoil the experience of enjoying a movie or having dinner in a cozy restaurant. You may find you have to ride a bicycle because you can no longer drive at night. Another common so-called minor side-effect is double or even triple vision and seeing starbursts around bright objects.

The American Food and Drug Administration (FDA) expects 10 percent of people who have undergone refractive surgery to be dissatisfied with the result. The FDA also expects 20 percent of them to lose low contrast acuity. Up to 15 percent of laser patients are expected to require enhancements or corrective surgery, frequently leading to additional costs.

The older and now less popular radial keratotomy (or microsurgery) consists of making a series of small incisions around the center part of the eye. The closer the incisions to the central optical zone, the greater the effect. This procedure actually inflicts open wounds on the cornea. The natural stress patterns of the cornea cause the wounds to open up in order to equalize the surface stress. Since healing takes many months the risk of infection is quite high. Also, the results are less predictable than with more modern laser treatment.

Even more serious, there is legislation under way in the United States and Canada which will prohibit people who have had laser surgery from driving at night. There is mounting evidence that the treatment causes a loss of the ability to distinguish details in low light and under backlit conditions. For example, it is easy to see the features of someone's face when they stand against a sunlit window. After laser surgery some individuals will only be able to see the outline, no longer being able to make out the details. In some cases people may also see halos around bright objects, making driving at night very dangerous. Refractive surgery has been added to the list of risk factors after the U.K. Transportation Research Laboratory tested myopics who had laser surgery and discovered that 80 percent of them could not see a traffic sign at 55 meters. Even worse, 40 percent could not see the sign at 15 meters (i.e., the length of four cars). In August 2000 the Canadian Medical Association added refractive surgery to the list of risk factors in unsafe driving.

Many people who have undergone microsurgery or laser treatment find that they have merely changed their near-sight glasses for a pair of reading glasses. A lot of the people who attend my Vision Training classes have had refractive surgery of one kind or another. They come because their vision is beginning to revert to where they were before the surgery. Remember, the fact is that you are still near-sighted even after you've had your surgery. The actual condition of your eye that meant you had near-sight is still the same. What has happened is that part of the cornea has been shaved off, thus altering the focus of the eye. In effect, the lenses have been actually carved onto your eyes. It is really just a step further than wearing contact lenses.

If you want to know what can happen after refractive surgery visit www.surgica-leyes.org. This website is well-balanced and informative, with lots of articles and personal stories about what can and does go wrong with refractive surgery. A wise ophthalmologist says that refractive surgery should be the last resort. In the same way we thought that breast implants were safe, we do not know what will happen 10 or 20 years after laser surgery. The FDA only approved the most popular procedure, LASIK, in 1998 (see www.fda.gov\LASIK).

Since there is so much hype and disinformation about laser treatment, I have compared excerpts from the FDA's LASIK surgery checklist with Vision Training.

Description	LASIK surgery	Vision Training
Know what makes you a poor candidate		
Career impact	Some employers prohibit laser surgery	N.A.
Cost	Between €1,500 to €3,000 per eye	Workshop costs €350
Medical condition	Illness that slows or alters healing	N.A.
Stable vision	Your vision must be stable for one year	N.A.
Pupil size	If your pupils are larger than 5.5 mm at night then you will experience starbursts	N.A.
Corneal thickness	Surgery not possible	N.A.
Dry eyes	Laser treatment aggravates dry eyes	N.A.

You may need more than one procedure to achieve the result you want		N.A.
You may still need reading glasses		N.A.
Results may not be long lasting		Results tend to last
You may experience permanent loss of vision		N.A.
You may not be able to drive at night	The FDA estimates that 20 percent of people lose contrast sensitivity making it impossible to see in dim light, such as restaurants, movie theaters, etc.	N.A.

You may experience halos and starbursts	Some people experience permanent double or triple vision effects	N.A.
Do not expect to see clearly for a few days	The final result may take months to materialize	You experience steady progress
Some people experience ghost images as in poor TV reception		N.A.
Expect some pain and discomfort	Expect to use eye drops to numb the pain	N.A.
Complications include irregular astigmatism	If the flap is wrinkled as a result of poor surgical procedure	N.A.
Corneal ectasia can develop	Due to the unavoidable thinning of the corneal tissue, the cornea can bulge out due to the internal eye pressure	N.A.

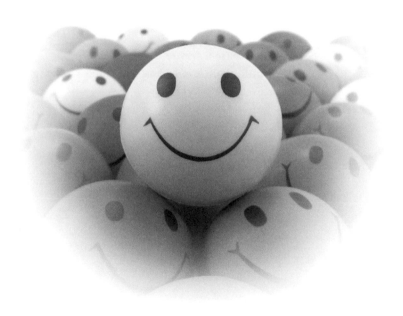

28. Your Vision Training Plan

Check your eyesight	Place the enclosed eye-chart on a wall in good daylight. Measure out the 1, 2 and 3 meter points from the chart. Check your visual acuity from 3 meters with both eyes.
Visual acuity of both eyes	What is the lowest line at which you can see and name the letters correctly? Note the 20/?? (printed on the right hand side of the eye-chart).
Visual acuity of left eye	Cover your right eye with your right hand. What is the lowest line at which you can see well enough to name the letters? Note the 20/??.
Visual acuity of right eye	Cover your left eye with your left hand. What is the lowest line you can see well enough to name the letters? Note the 20/??. If you have more than -5 diopters of myopia then you need to do the string measurement described on page 124.
Far point left eye	Measure the distance from the end of the string to the far point of the left eye in centimeters.
Far point right eye	Measure the distance from the the end of the string to the far point of the right eye in centimeters. Notice if there is a difference. If so then you need to work at educating both eyes to have the same far point.
Check for astigmatism	Look at the astigmatic mirror on page 92 and take in the overall image. If you notice that any of the lines are thicker, or are spaced closer or further apart, then you have an astigmatism. Be sure to check at different distances and test each eye as well.

Check eye-co-ordination   Use a string as described on page 151. You should see a phantom cross right through the paperclip at any distance within your visual range.

Astigmatism

● Do the Tibetan wheel exercise as described on page 94.

Near sight less than 2 diopters (you have clear vision out to 50 cm)

● Wear glasses only when absolutely necessary such as when driving.

● Work with the eye-chart as described on page 110.

● Practice the swinging exercises as described on pages 111 and 112.

● Make it a habit to search for the smallest possible object you can make out at the greatest distance.

● Do this exercise if you wish to practice with your contact lenses in.

Near sight between 2 and 3 diopters (your vision is somewhere between 37–50 cm)

● Don't use your glasses for reading and use them only when necessary.

● Do the string exercise described on page 124 to move your far point out.

● Practice with the chart-shifting exercise described on page 114.

● Play with the domino exercise on page 116.

● When you get closer to 2 diopters start doing the eye-chart exercise on page 110.

Near sight more than 4 diopters (you have clear vision only up to 25 cm)

● Wear lenses that are 0.5 to 0.75 diopter lower than your prescription.

● Do the energy exercise described on page 121.

● Do the string exercise described on page 124.

Eye co-ordination

● Work with the string as described on page 124.

Hyperopia

● Relax the eyes by using palming or by alternating hot and cold compresses.

- Exercise your ability to look at very small things very close-up.

- Don't wear plus lenses unless absolutely necessary.

- Read small print up-close and as often as possible.

Presbyopia

- Bring your near point of clear vision up to about 15 cm from both eyes.

- Reduce your prescription if necessary.

- Do the reading smaller and smaller print exercise on page 136.

- Practice the lazy reading exercise on page 141.

- Check your eye co-ordination with the circle exercise on page 142.

- Start reading without glasses in the morning when there is good daylight.

Amblyopia

- Do the string exercise with the lazy eye on page 124.

- Do the energy exercise described on page 121.

Strabismus

- Do the butterfly exercise on page 160.

- Do the long body swing on page 161.

- Do the mirror exercise on page 162.

Training your color perception

- Count colors as described on page 176.

- Match colors as described on page 177.

- Work with colors as described on page 177.

- Arrange colors as described on page 180.

The visually impaired

- Gaining light perception see page 182.

- Mapping across the senses see page 182.

- Gaining object recognition see page 183.

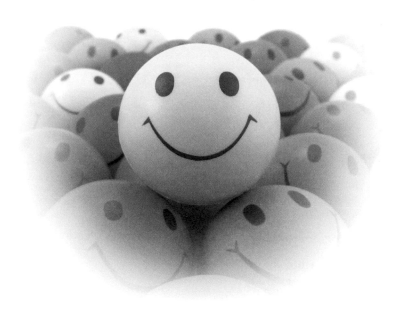

Appendix: The Science of Vision Training

The capacity to achieve substantial improvement in unaided visual acuity is well documented by, among others the American Optometric Association (1988). Early research was conducted by:

Bates (1920); Ewalt (1945); Woods (1946); Hildreth et al. (1947); Marg (1952); Epstein et al. (1978; 1981); Collins et al. (1981; 1982); Baillet (1982); Gil and Collins (1983); Blount et al. (1984); Rosen et al. (1984) and Berman et al. (1985).

The science of astigmatism

Over the years a number of researchers have come up with various theories about what causes astigmatism. The eminent German scientist Helmholtz (1909) suggested that due to anatomical factors, the eye would be expected to have against-the-rule astigmatism, but this tendency is countered by eyelid pressure, which tends to cause with-the-rule astigmatism. Duke-Elder (1932) suggested that with-the-rule astigmatism was related to the fact that the vertical diameter is slightly larger than the horizontal diameter.

Duke-Elder (1970) suggested that lid pressure could cause or alter corneal astigmatism. Vihlen and Wilson (1983) found that both with-the-rule astigmatism and the elastic coefficient of the lid decline with age, but they found no evidence that corneal torridity was determined by lid tension. Wilson et al. (1982) showed that lifting the eyelids reduced the corneal curvature in the horizontal meridian. They concluded that lid pressure did indeed produce some with-the-rule astigmatism, but generally, lifting the eyelids had little effect on corneal curvature when astigmatism was between 1 diopter with-the-rule or 1 diopter against-the-rule.

Pressure exerted by the extraocular muscles

A number of authors, including Fairmaid (1959), Bannon (1971) and Millodot and Thibault (1985), have reported that convergence of the eyes is accompanied by a falling of the horizontal corneal meridian, bringing about a slight increase in with-the-rule astigmatism or a decrease in against-the-rule astigmatism. Bannon (1971) estimated that the decrease in power of the horizontal corneal meridian accompanying convergence is from 0.245 to 0.5 diopters in non-presbyopic eyes.

Hofsteller and Rife (1953) concluded that astigmatism was mostly an environmentally determined trait. Lyle (1965) said that no hereditary patterns were discernible for astigmatism under 2 diopters.

Rigid contact lenses

Rigid contact lenses not only neutralize a portion of corneal astigmatism but often, with the passage of time, cause the cornea to become more toroidal. For example, wearing a flatter than normal contact lens in an attempt to reduce myopia (also known as orthokeratology) produces variable effects on corneal toricity, often including increased with-the-rule astigmatism. The development of with-the-rule astigmatism associated with the wearing of rigid contact lenses has been reported by many authors including Grosvenor (1977). The amount of astigmatism induced by polymethylmethacrylate (PMMA) lenses is reported to be from 2.5 to 6 diopters.

Residual astigmatism

Residual (internal astigmatism) refers to that part of the total astigmatism not attributed to the cornea. Residual astigmatism is against-the-rule astigmatism for most people (Neumueller, 1953) found 87 percent of the people he tested had against-the-rule astigmatism. Researchers found residual astigmatism between 0.5 and 0.75 diopters (Carter, 1972).

Researchers have mainly been interested in describing the phenomena of astigmatism. Only a few have suggested that the extraocular muscles may be involved in creating the corneal distortion typical of this condition. The Vision Training approach assumes that the exterior eye muscles, primarily the rectus muscles, are involved in distorting the cornea. This is not such a big leap of the imagination, since it is well known that the wearing of hard contact lenses leads to astigmatism.

The science of myopia

Myopia is the eye condition that has been studied more than any other. Interestingly enough, glasses were discouraged during the first half of the 1800s for myopia (MacKenzie, 1830) and for hyperopia (Sichel, 1837).

Is the prevalence of myopia related to the level of education?

The conclusion of early investigators (Cohn, 1867; Dor, 1878; Florchutz, 1880; von Jaeger, 1861; Ware, 1813) was that children in more intensive educational environments exhibited a higher prevalence of myopia. This finding was corroborated in a study of native Melanesian children (Garner, 1988), which showed a significantly higher prevalence among those who were involved in intensive study than those who were not.

Bind (1950) found almost no myopia among Eskimo children. Skeller (1959) reported that myopia was exceptionally rare among all Eskimos. However, in 1969 Young et al., reported that virtually no myopia existed among parents and grandparents, while more than half of the children of school age were myopic.

The ever increasing academic requirements for children is reflected by Sato (1957), where the prevalence of myopia increased from 15 percent in 1914 to an incredible 45 percent in 1955, when records of middle school children in Japan were examined.

Rosner and Belkin (1987) conducted a nationwide survey in Israel noting the degree of myopia and intelligence scores among 157,748 males aged between 17 and 19 years. This represented a largely unselected study population since all Jewish males of this age undergo medical examinations to check their fitness for military service. They found that both "years of schooling" and "intelligence" weighted approximately equally in their positive correlation with myopia.

Is the prevalence of myopia increasing?

Scheerer (1928) and Betsch (1929) examined 25,000 adults over the age of 25 and found that 13.7 percent of them had myopia. Walton (1950) examined 1,000 people aged between 30 and 90 and found 17.7 percent had myopia. British statistics from 2001 indicate that 61 percent of the population had myopia. Unfortunately, myopia appears to be increasing at an alarming rate.

At this point scientists do not know why myopia develops. There are many theories attempting to explain this, ranging from genetic disposition to simple over-use of the eyes for near work.

Does excessive near work lead to myopia?

Gross and Zhai (1994) propose a hypothetical mechanism explaining the development of myopia. They suggest that an individual who does a great deal of close work and who has a larger than normal lag of accommodation, and therefore a degraded retinal image, will be prone to myopia. This is because the lag of accommodation/ focusing places the image formed by the optical system behind the retina. As a result, the axial length increases, having the effect of placing the image clearly on the retina.

Continued near work could cause the axial length to increase. This process is hypothesized to operate in the same way as the normal emmetropizising mechanism. Some researchers refer to this as emmetropization at the near point.

Gwiazda et al. (1993) suggest that in an individual who has poor accommodation, the blurred images – not the accommodative effect – are the cause of myopia. Accommodative responses were measured for newly myopic and emmetropic (normal vision) children under three conditions. In the first situation, the stimulus to accommodate or focus was increased by moving the target closer (therefore simulating proximally induced accommodation); in the second condition the stimulus to accommodate was increased by the use of concave lenses; and in the third condition the stimulus to accommodation was decreased by the use of convex lenses.

When convex lenses were used to decrease the stimulus to accommodation, there was essentially no difference in accommodative lag for the two groups of subjects. When accommodation was stimulated by moving the target closer to the subject, the mean lag of accommodation was similar for the myopes and emmetropes at all but the closest distance of 25 cm, where the lag for the myopes was 0.4 diopters greater than for the emmetropes. However, when concave lenses were used to increase the stimulus to accommodation, the lag of accommodation was significantly greater for the myopes. A -3.50 diopter lens (the highest power used) read approximately 2.7 diopters for the myopes as compared to 1.5 diopters for the emmetropes.

Gwiazda et al., suggest that "reduced accommodation is found for a period after, and perhaps before, the onset of myopia, at whatever age it occurs" (1993: 693).

Experimentally induced myopia

The environment has a great influence on vision. For example, laboratory monkeys are found to be considerably more myopic than wild monkeys, and monkeys kept indoors in cages develop more myopia than animals kept in outdoor pens (Young, 1967).

The German researcher Levinson was the first person to conduct animal experimentation. Levinson believed that myopia resulted from the pull of the optic nerve when the eyes are held in a downward position, so that the anterior–posterior axis of the globe is oriented vertically. To test the theory, monkeys were placed in a box that was parallel to the floor, with the result that after a few months, myopia was found to occur and increased as long as the experiments were carried on. Griswell and Gross (1983) kept three monkeys in this position. One of them developed 14 to 15 diopters of myopia after nine months, the second developed 7 to 9 diopters of myopia after one year, and the third developed 1 to 2 diopters of myopia after four weeks. Intraocular pressure did not increase during the experiment and the myopia was axial in nature; in other words, the eyeball elongated in a way that is typical of myopia.

The science of convergence

Numerous clinical studies report on the efficacy of Vision Training for convergence insufficiency. Cooper and Duckman (1978) reviewed 15 studies of Vision Training for convergence insufficiency over a 47 year period. These studies surveyed nearly 2,000 patients and reported an overall cure rate of 72 percent, with improvement in an additional 19 percent, and failure in only 9 percent of cases.

Impressive cure rates are reported by Duthie and Mayou (1945), who achieved cures in 72 percent of 364 patients with convergence insufficiency.

The science of strabismus

Usually strabismus is managed by means of prism lenses or corrected by surgically weakening or tightening the eye muscles. Often there is immense pressure placed on parents to give permission for their children to undergo surgery. However, the result of strabismus surgery is not impressive. In many cases it is only a cosmetic procedure which fails to achieve stereoscopic vision.

Efficacy of the non-surgical Vision Training approach

Wick (1987) did a retrospective examination of the records of 54 patients who had undergone vision treatment for accommodative esotropia (the eye turning inwards). The patients were classified based on the Duane classification as having either convergence excess (n = 11) or equal eso-diversions (n = 43).

Over 90 percent of the patients achieved total restoration of normal binocular function with this treatment approach.

Chryssanthou (1974) studied 27 patients with intermittent exotropia (one eye turned out) with ages ranging from 5 to 33 years of age. A total of 89 percent of patients showed definite improvement, with 66.6 percent graded excellent six months to two-and-a-half years after treatment.

Etting (1978) reported a 65 percent overall success rate in patients with constant strabismus, specifically, 57 percent for esotropes (eye turning in) and 82 percent for exotropes (eye turning out). There was an impressive 89 percent success rate with intermittent strabismus, specifically, 100 percent of esotropes (eye turning in) and 85 percent of exotropes (eye turning out). Etting reported an astonishing 91 percent success rate when retinal correspondence was normal.

Flax and Duckman (1978) examined the effectiveness of orthoptics as a viable modality for treating strabismus. They reviewed the pertinent literature and presented an analysis of the data. The result of numerous studies showed a combined functional cure rate of 74 percent. Ludlam (1961) evaluated the efficacy of orthoptic strabismus treatment in a selected group of 149 selected strabismus sufferers who received Vision Training treatment, and determined a 73 percent overall success rate.

In a subsequent study Ludlam and Kleinman (1965) found the long-term success rate of vision therapy for strabismus to be 65 percent. Bryer (1961) investigated the long-term effects of treatment of heterophoria. Of 89 patients whose initial symptoms were completely relieved during treatment, 81 percent remained symptom free on follow-up six to ten years after treatment. Only 4 percent experienced a recurrence of symptoms severe enough to require further treatment. Also Vaegan (1979) reported successful results with isometric training in a 1979 study.

Many of the above studies may seem dated. However, the strabismic condition remains unchanged through time and the efficacy is thus still relevant and important.

The science of amblyopia

So far researchers have no understanding of the underlying causes of amblyopia. When amblyopia is associated with strabismus it is believed that the conflicting input from the two eyes results in active suppression and amblyopia of the non-dominant eye. Amblyopia may also be the result of stimulus deprivation caused by cataracts or by large hypermetropic errors.

Many researchers concentrate on the treatment and management of amblyopia. The prevailing belief is that the best possible vision in an amblyopic eye is obtained when the normal eye is prevented from seeing. Pugh (1954) found that vision decreases when both eyes are open, indicating that the normal eye has an inhibitory effect on the amblyopic eye. In a 1966 study, von Noorden and Leffler demonstrated that the greater the luminances of the stimulus to the normal eye the lower the vision in the amblyopic eye.

In some cases the normal eye becomes amblyopic after wearing patches. Ikeda (1980) demonstrated that stimulus deprivation of amblyopia could result from the use of atropine or penalization (wearing eye-patches).

Patching or penalizing the good eye was first recommended by de Buffon in 1743. This is still the preferred method of treatment by doctors to this day. Over the years attempts have been made to supplement this passive treatment with active stimulation of the eye. Electrical and chemical stimulation has been tried without much success.

The various strategies used are:

● Total occlusion, excluding all light and form. An example of this is placing adhesive occluders over the eyes. In some cases black contact lenses have been used.

● Total occlusion, excluding form but allowing some light. Examples of the treatment would be wearing frosted glasses or other filters.

- Partial occlusion, allowing the appreciation of form but diminishing its acuity. An example of this would be to cover only part of the eye. This partial occlusion is widely used in France. Another example is blocking the lower half of the lens to promote the use of the amblyopic eye for close work.

- Optical penalization uses lenses to blur the vision of the better eye in order to force the amblyopic eye to work.

- Cycloplegic drugs are used to blur the vision of the good eye. The drug commonly used is atropine as drops or ointment.

The prevailing medical approach is to force the amblyopic eye to work by blocking the vision of the good eye. Forcing small children to wear patches and in some cases actually restraining them by blocking elbow movements is fortunately becoming unacceptable to parents.

Causing the vision of the good eye to blur is also a questionable approach since it is well known that wearing lenses causes the eye to adjust to the lens worn. In this case the otherwise normal eye will be forced to lower its visual acuity as demonstrated by Ikeda and Tremain's (1978) research.

Bibliography

Papers

American Optometric Association (1988). Special report: the efficacy of optometric vision therapy. *Journal of the American Optometric Association*. 59: 95–105.

Balliet R., Clay A., Blood K. (1982). The training of visual acuity in myopia. *Journal of the American Optometric Association*. 53: 719–724.

Bailey I. L., Bullimore M.A. (1991). A new test of disability glare. *Optometry & Vision Science*. 68: 911–917.

Bannon, R. E., (1971). Near point binocular problems-astigmatism and cyclophoria. *The Ophthalmic Optician*. 11: 158–168.

Bates, W. H. (1915). The Cure of Defective Eyesight by Treatment Without Glasses. *New York Medical Journal*. 101 (19): 925–933.

Bates, W. H. (1918). A Study of Images Reflected from the Cornea, Iris, Lens, and Scler. *New York Medical Journal*. May 18.

Bates, W. H. (1922). Reading without glasses. *Better Eyesight* 6(2).

Bell C., Bell J., Davidson Godman J. (1827). *The Anatomy and Physiology of the Human Body*. 2: 227.

Berman, P. E., Levinger, S. I., Massath, N. A. et al. (1985). The effectiveness of bio-feedback visual training as a viable method of treatment and reduction of myopia. *J Optom Vis Dev*. 16: 17–21.

Betsch A. (1929). Uber die menschliche Refraktionskurve. Klzn. Mhl. Augenheilk. 82. 365–379.

Bind, E. (1950). Carrying optometrical services to the Eskimos of the eastern Artic. *American Journal of Optometry & Archives of the American Acadamy of Optometry.* 47: 24–31.

Blount et al. (1984). Improving visual acuity in a myopic child: Accessing compliance and effectiveness. *Behav Res Ther.* 22: 53–57.

Bryer, J. J. (1961). Assessment of the results of orthoptic treatment in herterophoria. *Br Orthopt J.* 18: 87–89.

Buffon, M. de (1743). Dissertation sur la cause du strabisme on les yeux louches. *Hist Acad R Sci.* 231–248.

Cohn, H. (1883). The Hygiene of the Eye in Schools. English translation by W. P. Turnbull, London: Simpkin, Marshall & Co, 54–55.

Chryssanthou, G. (1974). Orthopic management of intermittent exotropia. *Journal of the American Optometric Association.* 24: 69–72.

Coleman, D. J., (1969). Ophthalmic bimetry using ultra-sound. *International Ophthalmology Clinics.* 9: 667–683.

Collins, F. L., Epstein, L. H. and Hannay, H. J. (1981). A component analysis of an operant training program for improving visual acuity in myopic students. *Behavior Therapy.* 12: 692–701.

Collins, F. L., Ricci, J. A. and Burkett, P. A. (1982). Behavioural training for myopia: long term maintenance of improved acuity. *Behavior Research & Therapy.* 19: 265–268.

Cooper, J. and Duckman, R. (1978). Convergence insufficiency: incidence, diagnosis and treatment. *Journal of the American Optometric Association.* 49(6): 673–680.

Dalton, J. (1798). Extraordinary facts relating to the vision of colours. *Memoirs of the Literary Philosophical Society of Manchester.* 5: 28–45.

Dor, M. L. (1878). Etude sur l'hygiene oculaire au lycee de Lyon. Lyon Medical. Cited by Cohn, H.: Hygiene of the Eye. London: Simpkin, Marshall & Co. 1886.

Duke-Elder, S. (1932). The clinical significance of the ocular musculature: With special reference to the intra-ocular pressure and the circulation of the intra-ocular fluid. *Br J Ophthalmol.* 16(6): 321–335.

Duthie, O. M. and Mayou, S. (1945). The treatment of convergence deficiency. *British & Irish Orthoptics Journal.* 3: 72–82.

Elliot, D. B., Yang, K. C. H. and Whitaker, D. (1995). Seeing beyond 6/6. *Optometry & Vision Science*. 72: 186–191.

Epstein, L. H., Collins, F. L. and Hannay, H. J. (1978). Fading and feedback in the modification of visual acuity. *Journal of Behavioral Medicine*. 1: 273–287.

Epstein, L. H., Greenwald, D. J., Hennon, D. et al. (1981). Monocular fading and feedback: effects on vision changes in the trained and untrained eye. *Behavior Modification*. 5: 171–186.

Etting, G. (1978). Strabismus therapy in private practice: cure rates after three months of therapy. *Journal of the American Optometric Association*. 49: 1367–1373.

Ewalt, H. W. (1945). The Baltimore Myopia Control Project. *Journal of the American Optometric Association*. 17(5): 167–185.

Fairmaid J. A. (1959). The constancy of corneal curvature. *British Journal of Physiological Optics*. 16: 2–23.

Flax, J. and Duckman, R. (1978). Orthoptic treatment of strabismus. *Journal of the American Optometric Association*. 49: 1353–1361.

Florschutz, B. (1880). Die Kursichttigkeit in des coburger schulen, Coberg.

Garner, L. F., Kinnear, R. F., McKellar, M. et al. (1988). Refraction and its components in Melanesian schoolchildren in Vanuatu. *American Journal of Optometry & Physiological Optics*. 65: 182–189.

Gil, K. M. and Collins, F. L. (1983). Behavioural training for myopia: generalization of effects. *Behavioral & Research Therapy*. 21: 269–273.

Goldschmidt, E. (1968). On the etiology of myopia: an epidemiological study. *Acta Ophthalmol*. 98 (Suppl.): 1–172.

Greene, P. R. (1980). Mechanical considerations in myopia: relative effects of accommodation, accommodative convergence, intraocular pressure and extra-ocular muscles. *American Journal of Optometric Physiological Optics*. 47: 902–914.

Greene, P. R. (1981). Myopia and the extraocular muscles. *Doc Ophthal Proc Ser*. 28: 163–170.

Griswell, M. H. and Gross, D. A. (1983). Myopia development in experimental animals. *American Journal of Optometric Physiological Optics*. 60: 250–268.

Gross, D. A. (1988). Retinal image-mediated ocular growth as a possible etiological factor in juvenile-onset myopia. Vision Science Syposium, A Tribute to Gordon G. Heath. Indiana University, pp. 165–183.

Gross, D. A. (1994). Overcorrection as a means of slowing myopic progression. *American Journal of Optometric Physiological Optics*. 61: 85–93.

Gross, D. A. and Zhai, H. (1994). Clinical and laboratory investigations of the relationship of accommodation and convergence function with refractive error. A literature review. *Doc. Ophthalmol*. 86: 349–380.

Grosvenor, T. (1977). A longitude study of refractive changes between ages 20 and 40. Part 2: Changes in individual subjects. *Optom. Weekly*. 68: 455–457.

Gwiazda, J., Thorne, F., Bauer, J. and Held, R. (1993). Myopic children show insufficient accommodative response to blur. *Investigative Ophthalmology & Visual Science*. 34: 690–694.

Herman C. (1867). Undersuchung der Auge von 10,060 Schulkinder nebst Vorschlägen zur Verbesserung der den Augen nachtheiligen Schuleinrichtungen, eine ätiologische Studie. Lipzig: Urban und Schwartzenberg,

Hildreth, H. R., Mainberg, W. H., Milder, B. et al. (1947). The effect of visual training on existing myopia. *American Journal Ophthalmology*. 30: 1563–1576.

Hofsteller H. W., Rife D. C. (1953). Miscellaneous optometric data on twins. *American Journal of Optometry & Archives of American Academy of Optometry*. 30: 139–150.

Hurvich, L. M. and Jameson, D. (1957). An opponent-process theory of color vision. *Psychological Review* 64(6, Pt 1): 384–404.

Ikeda, H. (1980). Visual acuity, its development and amblyopia. *Journal of the Royal Society of Medicine*. 73.

Ingram, R. M., Walker, C., Wilson, J. M., Arnold, P. E., Dally, S. (1986). Prediction of amblyopia and squint by means of refraction at age 1 year. *British Journal of Ophthalmology*. 70(1): 12–15.

Jaeger von (1861). Uber die einstellung des dioptrischen aparatus im Menschlichen Auge. L.W. Seidel u, Sohn, U.V. Wasson Wien.

Kelly, C. R. (1962). The Creative Process, Vol. II Nos. 2&3 September 1962, Vancouver, WA, USA.

Kelly, T. S. B., Chatfield C., Tustein B., (1975). Clinical assessment of arrent myopia, *British Journal of Ophthalmology*. 59: 529–38.

Kerns, R. L. (1978). Research in orthokeratology. Part VIII: results, conclusions and discussion of techniques. *Journal of the American Optometric Association*. 49: 308–314.

Lam C. S. and Goh, W. S. (1991) The incidence of refractive errors among school-children in Hong Kong in relationship with the optical components. *Clinical and Experimental Optometry*. 74: 97–103.

Ludlam, W. M. (1961). Orthoptic treatment of strabismus. *American Journal of Optometry & Archives of American Academy*. 38: 369–388.

Ludlam, W. and Kleinman, B. (1965). The long range results of orthopic treatment of strabismus. *American Journal of Optometry & Archives of American Academy*. 42: 647–684.

Lyle, W. M., (1965). The inheritance of corneal astigmatism, Thesis (Ph.D.) Indiana University, 1965.

MacKenzie, W. (1830). A practical treatise on Diseases of the Eye. Longman, Rees, Orme, Brown & Green. Glasgow.

Mares-Perlman, J. A., Klein R., Klein, B. E. et al. (1996). Association of zinc and antioxidant nutrients with age-related maculopathy. *Archives of Ophthalmology*. 114: 991–997.

Marg, E. (1952). Flashes of clear vision and negative accommodation with reference to the Bates Method of visual training. *American Journal of Optometry & Archives of American Academy*. 29(4): 167–184.

Millodot, M. and Thibault, C. (1985). Variation of astigmatism with accommodation and its relationship with dark focus. *Ophthalmic and Physiological Optics*. 5: 297–301.

Neumueller, J. (1953). Optical, physiological and perceptual factors influencing the ophthalmometric findings. *American Journal of Optometry & Archives of American Academy*. 30: 281–291.

Noorden G. K., von Leffler M. B. (1966). Visual acuity in strabismic amblyopia under monocular and binocular conditions. *Archives of Ophthalmology*. 76(2): 172–177.

Pugh, M. (1954). Foveal vision in amblyopia. *British Journal of Ophthalmology*. 38: 321–328.

Raab E. (1982). Etionlogic factors in accommodative esotropia. *Transactions of the American Ophthalmological Society*. 80: 657–694.

Rayleigh, Lord (1881). On copying diffraction gratings and on some phenomenon connected therewith. *Philosophical Magazine*. 11: 196–205.

Rosen, R. C., Shiffman, H. R. and Meyers, H. (1984). Behaviour treatment of myopia: refractive error and acuity changes in relation to axial length and intraocular pressure. *American Journal of Optometry and Physiological Optics*. 61: 100–105.

Rosner, M. and Belkin, M. (1987). Intelligence, education, and myopia in males. *Archives of Ophthalmology*. 105: 1508–1511.

Rosner J. and Rosner J. (1989). The relationship between clinically measured tonic accommodation and refractive status in 6 – 14 year old children. *Optometry & Vision Science*. 66: 436–439.

Saladin, J. J., Usui, S. and Stark, L. (1974). Impedance cyclography as an indicator of ciliary muscle contraction. *Journal of the American Optometric Physiological Optics*. 51(9): 613–625.

Sato T., (1957). The Causes and Prevention of Acquired Myopia. Tokyo, Kanehara Shuppan Co. Ltd.

Scheerer, R. (1928). Zur enlwicklungsgeschectlichen Auffassung der Brechzustande des Auges. Ber. Zusammenkunft Dtsch. Ges. 47, 118.

Sheppherd, K. (1983). Personalities differ in visual systems. *Brain Mind Bulletin*. 8(16): 3.

Sichel, J. (1837). Revue trimestr. de la Clinique ophth., page 22.

Skeller E. (1954). Anthropological and ophthalmological studies on the Angmagssalik Eskimos. Meddelelser om Grenland. 107(4) 1:211.

Tamm, J., Tamm E., Rohn, J. W., (1992). Mechanism of Aging and Development. 62(2): 209–221.

Tokoro, T. and Kabe, S. (1985). Treatment of myopia and the changes in optical components. Report I: Topical application of neosynephrine and tropicamide. *Acta Soc Opthmol Japonicae*. 68: 1958–1961.

Tokoro, T. and Kabe, S. (1986). Treatment of myopia and the changes in optical components. Report II: Full- or under-correction of myopia by glasses. *Acta Soc Opthmol Japonicae*. 69: 140–144.

Vaegan. J. L. (1979). Convergence and divergence show large and sustained improvement after short isometric exercise. *American Journal of Optometry and Physiological Optics*. 56: 23–33.

Vaegan, J. L. and Taylor, D. (1980). Critical period for deprivation amblyopia in children. *Jpn J Ophthalmol*. 24: 241–250.

Vihlen and Wilson. (1983). The relation between eyelid tension, corneal toracity, and age. *Investigative Ophthalmology & Visual Science*. 24(10): 1367–7313.

Walton, W. G., (1950). Refractive findings of 1,000 patients from a municipal home for the indigent. *American Journal of Optometry & Archives of American Academy* of *Optometry*. 38(2): 149–160.

Ware, J. (1813). Observations relative to the near and distant sight of different persons. Phil. Trans. R. Soc. London. 103: 31–50. Watson, P. G., Sanac, A.S., Picketing, M. S. A comparison of various methods of treatment of amblyopia: a block study. *Trans.Ophthalmol*. Soc. (UK 1985); 104: 319–328.

Wick, B. (1987). Accommodative esotropia: efficacy of therapy. *Journal of the American Optometric Association*. 58: 562–566.

Wilson, G., Bell, C., Chotai, S. (1982). The effect of lifting the lids on corneal astigmatism. *American Journal of Optometry and Physiological Optics*. 59: 670–674.

Woods, A. (1946). Report from the Wilmer Institute on the results obtained in the treatment of myopia by visual training. *American Journal of Optometry & Archives of the American Academy of Optometry*. 29(4): 167–184.

Young, F. A. (1967). Myopia and personality. American *Journal of Optometry & Archives of the American Academy of Optometry*. 44(3): 192–203.

Young, F. A., Leary, G. A., Baldwin, W. R., West, D. C., Box, R. A., Harris, E. & Johnson, C. (1969). The transmission of refractive errors within Eskimo families. *Journal of the American Optometric Association*. 43: 676–685.

Young, Thomas. (1801). The Bakerian lecture on the mechanism of the eye.

Books

Abel, R. (1999). *The Eye Care Revolution*. New York: Kensington Publishing.

Agarwal, R. S. (1935). *Mind and Vision and Secrets of Indian Medicine*. Pondicherry, India: Sri Aurobindo Ashram Press.

Agarwal, R. S. (1971). *Yoga of Perfect Eyesight*. Pondicherry, India: Sri Aurobindo Ashram Press.

Barnes, J. (1990). *Improve Your Eyesight: A Guide To The Bates Method for Better Eyesight without Glasses*. London: Souvenir Press.

Bates, W. H. (1920). *Perfect Sight without Glasses*. New York: Central Fixation Publishing Co. (Later abridged, revised and republished as *Better Eyesight without Glasses*. New York: Henry Holt, 1943.)

Berschadsky, A. (2004). http://homepage.mac.com/omca/somca/ten_reasons.pdf (accessed December 5, 2011).

Benjamin, H. (1929). *Better Sight without Glasses*, 1st edn. Wellingborough: Thorsons.

Chaney, E. (1991). *The Eyes Have It: A Self-Help Manual For Better Vision*. New York: Instant Improvement.

Cohen, N. S. (1977). *Out Of Sight Into Vision: There Is More To Good Vision Than Reading Fine Print*. New York: Simon & Schuster.

Corbett, M. D. (1949). *Help Yourself To Better Sight*. Englewood Cliffs, NJ: Prentice-Hall.

Corbett, M. D. (1957). *A Quick Guide To Better Vision: How To Have Good Eyesight without Glasses*. Englewood Cliffs, NJ: Prentice-Hall.

Donders, F. C. (1864). *On the Anomalies of Accommodation and Refraction of the Eye*. Tr. W. D. Moore. London: New Sydenham Society.

Duke-Elder, S. (1966). *System of Ophthalmology*. Vol. X: Diseases of the Uveal Tract. Ed. H. Kimpton. St. Louis, MO: C.V. Mosby.

Duke-Elder, S. & Abrams, D. (1970): *Ophthalmic optics and refraction*. In: Duke-Elder. S, (ed). *System of Ophthalmology*. Vol 5. Kimpton, London.

Goodrich, J. (1986). *Natural Vision Improvement*. Berkeley, CA: Celestial Arts.

Goodrich, J. (1996). *Perfect Sight the Natural Way: How To Improve and Strengthen Your Child's Eyesight*. London: Souvenir Press.

Grinder, J. and Bandler, R. (1981). *Trance-formations: Neurolinguistic Programming and the Structure of Hypnosis*. Boulder, CO: Real People Press.

Grossmann, M. and Swartwout, G. (1997). *An Encyclopedia of Natural Eye Care*. New Canaan, CT: Keats Publishing.

Hackett, C. A. (1955). *Relax And See: A Daily Guide To Better Vision*. New York: Harper.

Helmholtz, H. von (1866). Handbuch der physiologischen Optik. Hamburg: L. Voss. (English translation in D. L. MacAdam, Sources of Color Science. Cambridge, MA: MIT Press, 1970.)

Helmholtz, H. Handbuch der physiologischen Optik, Ed. 3. 9. Kleczkowski: Post okul. 11: 9, 1909.

Hering, E. (1964). *Outlines of a Theory of the Light Sense*. Cambridge, MA: Harvard University Press.

Hoops, A. (1970). *Eye Power: Improved Self-Awareness, Vitality, and Mental Efficiency through Visual Training*. New York: Knopf.

Huxley, A. (1943). *The Art of Seeing*. London: Faber.

Kaplan, R. M. (1994). *Seeing without Glasses: Improving Your Vision Naturally*. Hillsboro, OR: Beyond Words Publishing Inc.

Kaplan, R. M. (1995). *The Power behind Your Eyes: Improving Your Eyesight with Integrated Vision Therapy*. Rochester, VT: Inner Traditions.

Lieberman, J. (1996). *Take Off Your Glasses and See*. Victoria, BC: Crown Publications.

McFadden, B. (1925). *Strengthening the Eyes: A System of Scientific Eye Training*. New York: McFadden Publishing.

MacFaydyn, R. J. (1958). *See Without Glasses*. New York: Fawcett (Premier).

Mansfield, P. (1997). *The Bates Method*. Time Warner, London: Alternative Health.

Markert, C. (1983). *Seeing Well Again without Glasses*. New York: Prentice-Hall.

Peppard, H. H. (1940). *Sight without Glasses*. New York: Garden City Books.

Price, C. S. (1934). *The Improvement of Sight by Natural Methods*, 1st edn. London. (Reprinted Cleveland, OH: Sherwood Press, 1946.)

Quackenbush, T. R. (1997). *Relearning to See*. Berkeley, CA: North Atlantic Books.

Rosanes-Berrett, M. (1991). *Do You Really Need Glasses*? New York: Station Hill Press.

Rosner, J. and Rosner, J. (1988). *Vision Therapy in Primary Care Practice: Procedures Manual*. Boston, MA: Butterworth Heinemann.

Index

A

accommodation 9–12, 100–102
    excessive 126
acuity: 39–45
    near-vision 43
acupressure 75, 77
acupuncture 14, 75, 78, 79
Agarwal, R. S. 13–14
Amblyopia 167–169
American Optometric Association 6
animal experiments 167
anisometropia 189
anomaloscope 174
astigmatic mirror 92
astigmatism: 16, 18, 91
    against-the-rule 89
    with-the-rule 89
atropine 10–12, 27, 212
anisometropic vision 126
Ashram, Sri Aurobindo 13

B

balance swing exercise 163
Bandler, Richard 1
Bates, William H. 3, 7, 8, 9, 12, 13, 22, 102
Bates Method 12, 13, 14, 73, 105, 146

belief change 67
belief strategy 64–67
beta-carotene 30, 31, 33, 35
bifocal glasses 13, 19, 129, 156
bioflavonoid(s) 36
blur circles 101
Bowman's layer 23, 24, 195
Brain Gym 169
Brown, Bennett 55
butterfly exercise 156, 158, 160, 203

C

calcium 37, 192
carotenoids 30
cataracts 13, 27, 33, 36, 192, 211
chart shifting exercise 113, 114, 202
Chinese medicine 75, 77
Chon, Herman 99
circle exercise 142, 203
coming and going exercise 126–128
cone cells 28–29, 30, 43, 47, 56, 134, 140, 171, 173, 174
contact lenses 103
contrast 42, 44
convergence 151
convergence practice exercise 153
Corbett, Margaret D. 12–13

D

decimal acuity 40–41
deuteranomaly 175, 176
deuteranopia 175
deuteranope 176
diet 30, 34, 35 *see also* nutrition
Dilts, Robert 67
diabetic retinopathy 28
diopter(s) 45
diplopia 150
divergence, *see* strabismus
dominant eye 70, 160
domino exercise 113, 116, 202
Donders, Franciscus Cornelius 9, 100, 129
double vision, *see* diplopia
driving 6, 28, 42, 43, 45, 49, 103, 185, 186, 189, 196, 197, 202

E

emmetropic 208
energy exercise 1, 123, 183, 202, 203
esotropia 150, 155, 160, 210
exotropia 150, 155, 156, 210
eye:
    cornea 23–24
    fovea 29–30, 35, 40, 123, 149
    iris 23, 27, 29
    lens 26–28
    macula 30–31, 33, 35
    muscles 21–23
    pupil 24
    recti 21–23
    retina 28
    structures 26, 47
    zonules 27

eye-chart:
    colored 107
    see also Snellen chart
eye patches 156, 168, 211, 212
eye swing 112

F

far-sight, *see* hyperopia
Finsen, Niels 191
fluorescent lighting 35, 43, 88, 134, 135

G

glaucoma 6, 13, 36, 37, 101
Goodrich, Janet 3, 13, 73, 164
Grinder, John 1, 2

H

Hackett, Clara 12–13, 159, 162, 181
Helmholtz, Hermann von 8–10, 100, 129, 171, 205
Hering, Ewald 172
heterophoria 155, 210
hue 172, 173, 174, 177, 179, 180
Huxley, Aldous 116
Hypermetropic 211
Hyperopia 145–147

I

illumination and contrast 42
imaginary eyes 71–72
improve distance vision exercise 186
internal vision 70
Ishihara Color Test 174

K

Kelly, Charles R. 72, 101
keratoconus 196

keratotomy; *see also* laser surgery

L

laser surgery 198
LASIK 6, 195, 197, 198, 200
lazy eye, *see* amblyopia
lazy reading exercise 141, 203
lenses:
    minus 18, 46, 69, 71, 106
    plus 18, 46, 71, 133, 145, 203
light perception 181, 182, 203
lutein 30, 31, 33, 34, 35

M

macular degeneration 6, 28, 31, 34
Mansfield, Peter 14
mapping 182, 203
meridian(s) 77–79, 89, 91, 205, 206
mirror swing exercise 162
mono-vision 136, 149, 189
multiple personality disorder (MPD) 55–56
myopia:
    functional 104
    structural 104, 106

N

near-sight, *see* myopia
near vision acuity 43
near vision test 43, 87
Newton, Iassac 171
night vision 6, 43
neuro-linguistic programming (NLP) 1–3, 62, 67
nutrition 33–37

O

object recognition 181, 183
oblique muscles 9–12, 22, 23, 102, 126, 127, 128
opponent color theory 172–173
ophthalmologist(s) 15, 89, 126, 130, 156
opponent color vision 172
optical dimensions 25
optometrist(s):
    behavioural 16
    functional 159
Orthokeratology 206
oxidative stress theory 33, 192
oxygen 37, 103

P

palming 3, 105, 114, 116, 123, 137, 146, 168, 182, 186, 202
percentage acuity 41
peripheral vision 47
photopia 193
photosensitive cells 29, 47, 173, 192
pinhole glasses 101
pranic healing 121
presbyopia 43, 87, 129–143, 146, 203
prescription 18–19
primary colors 29, 171, 177, 178, 182
prism(s) 19, 152–153, 155, 210
protanomaly 175–176, 179
protanopia 175–176

Q

Quackenbush, Thomas 13

R

radial keratotomy 196
reading light 43, 135
reality strategy 62, 64, 66
red–green sensitivity 173
retinoscope 8–9, 131–132
rod cells 28–9, 43, 134, 140
rohodosin 29–30

S

Samurai 112
Schlemm's canal 27
secondary colors 176, 178, 182
sensory alignment exercise 50
Sheppherd, Kenneth 54
small print exercise 136
smoking 36
Snellen, Hermann 42
Snellen acuity 42
Snellen chart 41, 84–85, 110, 136
stereoscopic vision, *see* convergence
strabismus 16, 145, 150, 153, 155–165, 203, 210
string exercise 46, 113, 119, 124–126, 150, 202, 203
submodalities 70
sunglasses 191–193
supplements 34–37, 192
swinging 110, 111, 113, 116, 161, 185, 186, 202

T

Tibetan wheel exercise 90, 93, 94, 126, 202
trichromatic color theory 171
tromboning 116

tromboning exercise 164

U

ultraviolet (UV) light 191, 192
under-correction 121, 218

V

vergence 44, 149
vision training 4, 5, 6–14
    plan 201–203
    principles for amblyopia 169
    principles for astigmatism 90–92
    principles for convergence 150–151
    principles for hyperopia 146–147
    principles for presbyopia 133–137
    principles for strabismus 159–160
visual impairment 181–183
vitamin A 33, 35, 43
vitamin B complex 35
vitamin B1 36
vitamin B2 36
vitamin B6 36
vitamin B12 36
vitamin C 27, 33, 34, 36, 37, 192
vitamin D 37, 192
vitamin E 37

Y

Young, Francis 59
Young, Thomas 101, 171
Young–Helmholtz theory 171, 207, 209

Z

zeaxanthin 30, 31, 33, 35

About the Author

Leo Angart was born in Denmark and has lived in Asia for more than 30 years. For most of that time he lived in Hong Kong. Currently he is based in Munich.

Leo wore glasses for more than 26 years before he discovered how to regain his normal eyesight in 1991. The remarkable thing about his recovery is that it was accomplished through methods outside the traditional vision improvement methods. Leo has combined his knowledge of neuro-linguistic programming with many years of experience helping people to regain their eyesight. He has distilled his methodology into simple exercises specific to particular problems. Most importantly, the exercises give quick results.

This book is especially written for people with the most common vision problems such as near-sight, far-sight, astigmatism, eye co-ordination problems, strabismus and amblyopia. In the Chinese population the prevalence rate of myopia has already exceeded the 80 percent level. Leo feels that something has to be done to reverse this trend. He says: "The solution to good eyesight is not found in optometry. Glasses only give the impression of correcting your vision, as you know you are still near-sighted when you take your glasses off. My approach to Vision Training will restore your vision to the natural clear sight nature intended you to have."

Since 1996 Leo has conducted his weekend Vision Training workshops more than 25 times every year in major cities around the world. His workshops fill up quickly because they provide the how of Vision Training. Leo will give you the motivation and the specific steps. You in turn are responsible for doing the exercises. The encouraging part is that you will see an improvement almost immediately.

In addition there is more information at www.vision-training.com.

If you would like to attend one of Leo's workshops, please check the schedule on the website to find a workshop near you.

Testimonials for Leo Angart's workshops

I enjoyed the workshop immensely and having previously got my vision down from -8ish to 5ish and becoming 'stuck' there I am looking forward to making the final step as I do believe that Leo has provided me with the missing keys re the exercise for astigmatism and, more especially, the pranic energy exercise.

Please keep me informed of workshops that I might find relevant.

Andina

Primarily I would like to thank you for organising Leo's natural vision workshop in London 3 weeks ago, for allowing me to attend at a reduced rate (much appreciated) but most of all for the fact that it was truly amazing: everything that I wished for and more. For this, my heartfelt thanks go, of course, to Leo as well as to yourself, so I would be grateful if you were able to forward my gratitude to him. I thought he led the sessions thoughtfully and gently, in perfect balance with his huge enthusiasm and great energy (and deep knowledge of the subject); considering this is such an emotional issue for so many of us, I felt held and respected as well as instructed ... I returned home revitalised and inspired, having brought back so many gifts from the two days ... and the manual, also, is truly a gem.

I can report that already, only two weeks after the workshop, having followed Leo's advice (doing energy work and the ,pen' exercise several times a day ... and the ,string' every morning), I visited my local contact lens specialist on Monday asking for a lower prescription because I felt my lenses had become too strong ... and, being met with a half-scared, half-incredulous stare by the optician, indeed I was found to be right because, to their amazement, they confirmed that my lenses had become too strong and my prescription has now been reduced from -6.50 in both eyes to -6.00 in both eyes! I can't tell you how victorious I felt going home with a pack of reduced strength contacts! It was wonderful.. and considering that only 2 years ago I was on -7.50 and -7.00 (R and L eye), it is a compounded improvement ...

I feel that Leo has given me a renewed sense of motivation and self-belief to continue along this road and persevere to achieve better and better natural vision. I know I can do it with patience and plenty of love.

Elisabetta

I enjoyed the workshop by Leo. Did you know that after the second session I went to buy new contact lenses, 0.5 less than what I usually wear? However, when I measured my eyes the next morning, my grade for my right eye was even lower!! I am now wearing 3.5 in both eyes. I am working to bring both my eyes to -3.0 by the end of September (I started with 4.5 for my right eye and and 4.25 for my left eye). Thanks!!

Ruth

I did the weekend workshop in October 08 when my eyes were -4.50. Now I am wearing -1.75 contacts which I feel are becoming clear so I will decrease next month. I am just doing the Pranic Healing meditation exercise 2 hourly now. I am happy to help out at the next workshop also.

Narelle

Just wanted to thank Leo for a wonderful and inspiring course. I have already received such wonderful benefits and I know I will be successful in regaining my vision.I feel the luckiest person on earth to have found you, as my head felt like it was under water for so long. To walk outside and see clearly for the first time in years was truly a miracle.Thank you for your humble and charming way of conducting the course and for having the sensitivity to help Lance - that made me cry all the way home. If you ever decide to run a course on teaching people to teach this I would be very honoured. You have given me the greatest gift. Thank you.

Andrea

I attended Leo's vision course at the weekend and it was brilliant. I just wanted to write to say thank you for coordinating such a wonderful course. I gained a lot of insight from it and will be telling all my friends about it.

I haven't had my lenses in for 2 days now and I am determined not to put them back in ever again.

Go Leo!!

Michelle

You may remember me. I'm the "Going to be commercial pilot in Melbourne", who was at your course in October 2008. I have finished all my theory courses and passed my Instrument rating and in another 4 - 5 weeks I will go for my commercial flight test, so things are moving. Now the best news is I went to the "Class One Medical examination" (this initial one is the hard one to pass), all is OK, and have it in writing that I don't need glasses for flying and/or map reading at night. They put some drops in my eyes and noted that I'm a bit long sighted but not to a degree that I require glasses, so I'll keep doing the excercises. I'm not yet at the candle light stage but I'm getting there ...

Peter

My daughter Ana and I were on your training in Slovenia in December. Ana has problems with strabismus, so she had glasses. Now she is without glasses and her eyes are OK.

Thank you for everything.

Metka

I was in the vision therapy group that finished last night, February 6. What a wonderful course this is. I've had no discernible difference in actual vision but my eyes are absolutely popping with excitement about the near future. No more specs! Ye ha!

Today I went searching for an optometrist to change my spectacle prescription to a lower range. The glasses I am now wearing hurt my eyes even before I did your course but the optometrist kept telling me it was because I would not allow myself to adjust to the bifocals and other equally insulting nonsense. I was most naive when I trotted off to the first optometrist to request the lowering of my lens prescription. Seventy five million optometrists later I can no longer lay claim to being naive. I've outright lied, thrown hissy fits, burst into tears (yeah, okay, I confess - it was crocodile tears but the situation was desperate), hopped up and down pretending to be a lunatic (I heard exactly what you thought then Leo Angart! Be nice.), even attempted what I felt to be a rather grand Her Majesty Queen Elizabeth impersonation. All of this after telling the simple truth had failed at the first sixty five million visits. No one will change the lens without first doing an eye test and this is a pointless exercise as I will merely end up again with the same prescription.

So, my question is … do you know of a Bogart type optometrist who will meet me at midnight on whatever corner specified and take charge of changing my specs? I promise on my honour not to spill to the Feds, to resist any and all torture and never, ever under any circumstances reveal your name. I suspect the Feds might be on to me anyway as my first two emails to you disappeared with absolutely no trace. I will protect your identity with fierce integrity.

Just to remind you about my prescription at present: (L) -3.00, (R) -4.25. Your suggestion was to change to -3.25, perhaps even -3 so it's really only one lens that needs to be changed - isn't it?? I think I've got it right, maybe not.

Susan

When you asked me, as we were finishing, what result I had achieved, I replied that I didn't seem to have any noticeable result yet. I was wrong. When I arrived home I tried on a pair of old reading glasses that didn't work for reading. AMAZINGLY THEY WORKED! So I did get an improvement!

I will be continuing with the program until I reach PERFECT EYESIGHT!

Thank you once again for a wonderful program!

Toby

I did Leo Angart's vision training in 2004. At the time I was wearing bifocals and had a significant astigmatism problem. I had worn glasses for over fifty years. I am an author and by 2004 I had authored or co-authored 14 books. This meant I spent many hours at my computer and continue to do so. I found that during the workshop my astigmatism was significantly less, but I still felt insecure so I continued to wear my glasses. I did the exercises I had learned in the course plus I throughly read Leo's book *Improving Your Eyesight Naturally*. After about 6 months I decided to bury my glasses. I found that continuing to do various exercises for a few minutes each day helped me maintain my improved eyesight. I had no trouble reading and driving and my astigmatism was gone. The time I now spend looking after my eyes is far less than the time I use to spend looking for my glasses!

Ysaiah